Sweet Potato Soul

Easy Vegan Recipes

Author

Beth A. Green

© Copyright 2021 by Beth A. Green -All rights reserved.

This document is geared towards providing exact and reliable information with regards to the topic and issue covered. The publication is sold with the idea that the publisher is not required to render accounting, officially permitted, or otherwise, qualified services. If advice is necessary, legal or professional, a practiced individual in the profession should be ordered.

- From a Declaration of Principles which was accepted and approved equally by a Committee of the American Bar Association and a Committee of Publishers and Associations.

In no way is it legal to reproduce, duplicate, or transmit any part of this document in either electronic means or in printed format. Recording of this publication is strictly prohibited and any storage of this document is not allowed unless with written permission from the publisher. All rights reserved.

The information provided herein is stated to be truthful and consistent, in that any liability, in terms of inattention or otherwise, by any usage or abuse of any policies, processes, or directions contained within is the solitary and utter responsibility of the recipient reader. Under no circumstances will any legal responsibility or blame be held against the publisher for any reparation, damages, or monetary loss due to the information herein, either directly or indirectly.

Respective authors own all copyrights not held by the publisher.

The information herein is offered for informational purposes solely, and is universal as so. The presentation of the information is without contract or any type of guarantee assurance.

The trademarks that are used are without any consent, and the publication of the trademark is without permission or backing by the trademark owner. All trademarks and brands within this book are for clarifying purposes only and are the owned by the owners themselves, not affiliated with this document.

Contents

- INTRODUCTION 6
- Part I 7
- CHAPTER 1 7
- DESIGNED FOR A DIFFERENT WORLD 7
- CHAPTER TAKEAWAY 13
- CHAPTER 2 13
- THE STORY OF THE LOWLY SWEET POTATO 13
- CHAPTER TAKEAWAY 21
- Part II 21
- CHAPTER 3 21
- CALORIES ARE NOT CREATED EQUAL 21
- CHAPTER TAKEAWAY 36
- CHAPTER 4 36
- HORMONES: MANAGING THE BODY'S TRAFFIC SIGNALS 36
- CHAPTER TAKEAWAY 47
- CHAPTER 5 47
- INFLAMMATION: WHEN FOOD BECOMES FOE 47
- CHAPTER TAKEAWAY 52
- CHAPTER 6 52
- ACTIVITY: MORE IS NOT ALWAYS BETTER 52
- CHAPTER TAKEAWAY 58
- Part III 58
- YOUR BODY, YOUR RULES 58
- CHAPTER 7 58
- A STEP-BY-STEP GUIDE TO OPTIMIZE YOUR HEALTH 58
  - RECALIBRATING OUR CARB-O-METER: COUNTING CARBS TO RESET NORMAL 64
  - OPTIMIZING CARBS: HOW YOU LOOK, FEEL, AND PERFORM TO REFINE CARB INTAKE 67
  - MY BODY'S RESPONSE TO ITS DIET: GLUCOSE TESTING END OF DAY CHECK-IN 73

WHAT FOODS WILL MAKE ME FAT: GLUCOSE TESTING RESPONSE TO FOODS 74

GET OFF THE SUGAR ROLLER COASTER: GLUCOSE TESTING THROUGHOUT THE DAY 75

ARE MY CELLS STILL LISTENING? AT HOME GLUCOSE SENSITIVITY TEST 77

THE BODY'S GLUCOSE TRACKER: HBA1C 80

LEARNING FROM CONTINUAL GLUCOSE MONITORING: DEXCOM IMPLANT. 81

HOW TO IMPROVE YOUR CHOLESTEROL IN TWO WEEKS WITHOUT DRUGS.. 92

LEARNING FROM A FAT-FILLED DIET: EXPERIMENTS IN KETOSIS 93

IS MY BODY INFLAMED? C-REACTIVE PROTEIN 100

IDENTIFYING PROBLEM FOODS: INTOLERANCE/ALLERGY STUDY 101

IS MY BODY STRESSED? DAILY CORTISOL PATTERN 103

CHOOSING THE ACTIVITY THAT IS RIGHT FOR MY BODY: CORTISOL RESPONSE TO EXERCISE 105

GET ON TOP OF YOUR HEALTH: THE GRAND DADDY OF BLOOD WORK; WELLNESSFX 109

CHAPTER TAKEAWAY 111

Part IV 112

CHAPTER 8 112

SWEET POTATO BASICS 112

CHAPTER TAKEAWAY 120

CHAPTER 9 120

PRIMAL RECIPES FOR A MODERN WORLD 120

   Morning Hash With Sweet Potato 121

   Braised Apples and Sweet Potato in Spiced Honey over Grainless Granola 122

   Braised Apples and Sweet Potato in Spiced Honey 123

   Grainless Granola 124

   Sweet Potato Linguine with Sage and Brown Butter Sauce 125

   Moroccan Spiced Chicken 127

   Salad with Roasted Chicken, Sweet Potato, and Shallots 128

   Halibut with Sweet Potato and Citrus 130

   Swordfish with Sweet Potato Salsa 131

   Stuffed Sweet Potato Three Ways 132

   Baked Yam 132

   Beef Sausage Filling for Baked Yam 133

- Pork Sausage Filling for Baked Yam 133
- Lamb Sausage Filling for Baked Yam 134
- Spicy Beef with Pepper and Sweet Potato 135
- Turkey Burger Cookies 137
- Hearty Vegetable Soup 137
- Sopa de Batata Doce 140
- Southwestern Chili 141
- One-Pan Scramble with Sweet Potato 143
- Sweet Potato Frittata 144
- Rainbow Cubes 146
- Sweet Potato Vegetable Latkes 147
- Sweet Potato Poppers 149
- Sweet Potato Slaw 151
- Dressing 152
- Spinach Salad with Sweet Potato, Bacon, Walnuts, and Pomegranates ... 153
- Chard with Sweet Potato, Pine Nuts, Golden Raisins, and Prosciutto ... 155
- Grilled Sweet Potato with Lime and Cilantro Dressing 157
- Sweet Potato Mash Three Ways 158
- Sweet Potato Prep 158
- Mashed Sweet Potato with Orange and Ginger 158
- Okinawa Mash 159
- Whipped Yams with Caramelized Apples 159
- Oven-Roasted Winter Vegetables 161
- Sweet Potato Gratin Stackers 162
- Vegetable Tian 163
- On-the-Go Sweet Potato Quiche 165
- Spicy Sliced Sweet Potato 167
- Sweet Potato Bars 168
- Fudge Brownie Bites 169
- Chocolate Sweet Potato Truffles 171
- Sweet Potato Ice Pops 173
- Sweet Potato Cupcakes 174
- Recovery Drink 176
- About the Supplements 176

Sport Gels Three Ways 177

INTRODUCTION

Carbohydrate-conscious diets are here to stay. While many people believe that low-carb diets are a passing trend, the idea of limiting carbohydrates has been around for centuries. When Tolstoy wrote Anna Karenina in 1873, one of his characters made explicit reference to the power of low-carb diets. Anna's lover, Count Vronsky, "avoided starchy foods and dessert" to lean out for an upcoming horse race. Countless books about low-carb diets have rehashed and modified the concept.

Recently the paleo diet, focusing on foods our biology was designed to consume, has emerged as a refined version in the low-carb world. Instead of the amount of carbs (low vs. high), the diet emphasizes the quality of carbohydrates—vegetables, some starch, and little fruit—and eliminates health culprits, such as grains, legumes, and high-carb processed food.

With the paleo diet, food has once again become a powerful drug in the arsenal of health. Patients have been cured of diabetes. Prediabetics have taken control of their diets so they do not need medical intervention. Markers for heart diseases have disappeared. Autoimmune disease is brought under control. Overweight men and woman lean out. People are coming out of their diet-induced mental fogs—regaining energy in body and mind. Kids are less prone to temper tantrums. And athletes are seeing gains in their performance. Individual by individual, the merits of this way of life are spreading and becoming mainstream.

So, what does a carb-conscious diet have to do with sweet potatoes? The answer is simple. For all of the benefits of a paleo diet, it can leave you feeling depleted, as if there is not enough gas in the tank, while at the same time requiring the constant eating of low-energy, dense foods. A sweet potato is a smart carb—a nutritionally-packed food source that gives your cells the energy they need without the negative side effects that accompany other energy-dense foods, such as wheat, rice, and corn. Sweet potatoes can be a powerful ally in our efforts to eat primal in a modern world.

Beyond the story of the humble sweet potato (a smart carb all-star that is often underappreciated and underutilized), this book arms you with easy-to-understand nutritional science in order to make the right choices for your specific body and lifestyle. It explains how your body deals with food, provides easy to follow instructions for tracking important health markers, and equips you with the tools to administer and interpret your own tests.

We were not meant to follow the same diet. Each of us has our own blueprint for optimal health. How do we get this new understanding? The answer is data—data from your body based on your biology. Your own data will cut through the conflicting opinions. The tools are available. This book describes the tools and provides the knowledge of how to use them. You can learn to speak the language of your own unique body and come to your own conclusions. Your body. Your rules.

The tests and monitoring described in this book will also give you the ability to listen to your body for warning signs, so that you can make the necessary lifestyle changes to avoid disease and chronic health conditions. That personal narrative is all we need to cut through the health noise around us and make better choices. Now that is powerful stuff.

Once you understand what your body can and cannot tolerate, you will be able to utilize sweet potatoes—nature's gem—to full advantage. Sweet potatoes will provide you with consistent energy throughout the day, the ability to demand superior mental and physical performance from your body and mind, the fuel to engage in extended activities, and the nutrients your cells need for faster recovery between workouts. With sweet potatoes you can do what you love without compromising the benefits of a carb-conscious lifestyle. And, to top it all off, sweet potatoes are a delicious addition to any meal!

Part I

SMART CARBS

NUTRITIONAL STARVATION IN THE ERA OF SUPERMARKETS, AND WHY THE SWEET POTATO DESERVES A SUPERSTAR SPOT ON THE TABLE

CHAPTER 1

DESIGNED FOR A DIFFERENT WORLD

FOOD TECHNOLOGIES HAVE CHANGED; OUR BODIES HAVE NOT

The Way We Were versus the Way We Are Now

Human DNA, our body's manual for interpreting everything it encounters, evolved millions of years ago in a world drastically different from our own. Our primal ancestors worked hard for the food they ate. With only basic tools and fire, they successfully hunted animals, collected and prepared wild vegetables, and destroyed deadly microbes by cooking and preserving their meals. Over time, evolution designed their bodies to thrive on the food that was available in their environment.

Survival required energy-rich fat to fuel activity, seasonal sugar to add extra fat stores for winter, and the occasional mineral salt to balance fluids in the body. But the varying availability of foods meant these necessities were not always around. When they were available, our ancestors had to take advantage and eat up. Gorging in a time of plenty was valuable genetic programming that would save them in a time of scarcity.

No one can tell the stories of these isolated people better than the diligent researchers who studied and recorded the changes within these isolated populations as Western diets were introduced. Such individuals include George Catlin among the Plains Indians; John Rae, Frederick Schwatka, and Vilhjalmur Stefansson among the Inuit; John Orr and J. L. Gilkes among the Masai; and Staffan Lindeberg among Kitavans. Their firsthand accounts make for fascinating reading. If you are interested in learning more on the topic, here are some good books to digest:

Nutrition and Physical Degeneration
by Weston A. Price

Food and Western Disease, Health and Nutrition from an Evolutionary Perspective
by Staffan Lindeberg

Physiological and Medical Observations among the Indians of Southwestern United States and Northern Mexico
by Ales Hrdlicka

Modern Food Technology—Not as Good as Nature's Complexity

Take a bite of a ripe, juicy, heirloom tomato. Flavors dance in your mouth as the juiciness explodes. Compare this experience to a store-bought tomato. A bite does not melt; it crunches, or worse, dissolves into mealy blandness. Flavors fall flat. Tomatoes and other seasonal produce are now made available year-round, thanks to farmers and food scientists. While they appeal to our eyes in the market, our taste buds don't rejoice with their diminished flavor.

Today, decisions about what to grow are based on maximizing yield, shelf life, ease of shipping, and storing. What is produced and sold is what is commercially viable. What is commercially viable is not always the healthiest or best tasting. Commercial farmers replace compost, nature's fertilizer, with synthetic fertilizers full of nitrogen, potassium, and phosphorus because it produces high yields. But plants need much more to thrive. In this case quantity replaces quality. Despite greater yields, soil is depleted and our foods don't contain the complexity of nutrients they once gained from nature's richness. Just take the difference between a store-bought tomato and the real thing. Taste—and nutrients—are lost when we tinker with nature's complexity.

The same can be said for the way we treat our foods in order to extend shelf life. We actually remove nutrients from many foods to allow them to keep longer. For example, flour used to be a perishable food. Then, somebody figured out that we could remove the nutrients ("germ") that critters like to eat, making flour last longer. This technology made flour a commercially viable product, but at the expense of the nutrients it originally contained. And what is done with the stripped nutrients from wheat? It's added to smoothies or other "nutritional" supplements!

We created all this technology to make food grow all the time, regardless of season, and last longer. It doesn't mean that we have a solid understanding of food science. We supposedly know more about food than ever before—but where has all this understanding of science and food technology gotten us?

The Paleo Diet: A Tool to Help Identify the Foods Our Bodies Were Meant to Consume

As bad food technologies continue to sneak into the most innocent of food sources, many people have decided to turn to the foods of our ancestors of the Paleolithic period, the earliest period of the Stone Age, in order to avoid the unhealthy choices that pervade the modern food industry. A paleo diet focuses on the foods that our bodies are most likely to thrive on after hundreds of thousands of years of evolution. They are the foods our hunter-gatherer ancestors ate: wild animals, fish, foraged vegetables, and seasonal fruit.

A paleo diet tries to closely mimic the diet of our ancestors using the guideline: meats, vegetables, nuts, seeds, some starch, little fruit, and no sugar. This regimen has helped thousands regain control of their health and body and reverse chronic disease. Devoid of grain, refined sugars, legumes, and dairy, paleo diets are nutritionally dense on a calorie-for-calorie basis. The following books are worth a read for a detailed discussion of the diet:

The Paleo Solution: The Original Human Diet
by Robb Wolf

The Primal Blue Print
by Mark Sisson

The Paleo Diet
by Loren Cordain, Ph.D.

Frankenfoods and Technology Gone Awry

Technological food innovations can be good (beneficial) or bad (harmful). Using fire to kill microbes is good. Irradiating to increase shelf-stabilization is bad, as it destroys the nutrients along with microbes. Drying and curing to sustain food's longevity is good. Refined vegetable oils that add to shelf life are bad. Meat with a side of vegetables is good. A bar to replace a meal is bad. Good technology helps us prepare and cook foods, adds to the diversity of foods we eat, and helps us to carry food on-the-go. Modern food processing methods strip nutrients from foods and leave us with food imposters that degrade our health.

In the last few decades, we have been given Frankenfoods—monster-like creations stitched together using various modern technologies in an attempt to create the most ideal commercially viable foods. Zap for shelf stabilization. Spray with vitamins for better nutritional labeling. Enhance taste with artificial flavors. Alter textures with additives. Entomb in plastic to lengthen shelf life. The result: a monster, the Frankenfood.

Today these Frankenfoods crowd our supermarket shelves and make up the bulk of the civilized world's diets. But these technologies are not the technologies that best serve our well-being. If we want to optimize our health and performance, we need to eat as we were programmed to eat.

Fossilized sweet potatoes from 10,000 years ago were found in Peru.

Good Food Processing Technologies

....

COOKING

Preparing food by the process of heat. Kills or deactivates potential harmful organisms, such as bacteria or viruses. Destroys antinutrients in some plants and improves digestibility.

DRYING

Method of food preservation by removing water from food via evaporation (air drying, sun drying, smoking, or wind drying).

SMOKING

Process of adding flavor, cooking, or preserving foods by exposing them to burning or smoldering plant material.

SALTING

Process of preserving foods by adding edible salt. Kills most bacterial fungi and other pathogenic organisms.

FERMENTING

A controlled anaerobic breakdown of energy-rich compounds, such as carbohydrates, using yeasts and bacteria.

STORING

Action or method of storing for further use in dry, cool spaces, including cellars and mounds.

Bad Food Processing Technologies

....

IRRADIATION

Process by which a food is exposed to radiation in order to sterilize. It not only strips food of bacteria and viruses, but also zaps nutrients.

PASTEURIZATION

Process of heating foods to a certain temperature for a specified period of time. Used to slow microbial growth to extend the shelf life. Destroys enzymes and beneficial microbes.

ADDITIVES

Substances added to food to enhance flavor and/ or appearance and/or shelf life. Food additives include anti-caking agents, antifoaming agents, antioxidants, bulk agents, food coloring, color retention agents, emulsifiers, flavors, flavor enhancers, glazing agents, preservatives, stabilizers, sweeteners, and thickeners.

FORTIFICATION

Process of adding micronutrients to foodstuffs. Food producers add or spray nutrients destroyed in the stabilization process that are thought to be healthy. However, as in the case of folic acid, these substances that are intended to bolster the health of a food can be harmful.

PLASTIC PACKAGING

Enclosing or protecting products for storage, large-scale distribution, and sale. (When food is brought to high temperatures, as in a microwave, plasticizers in the plastics can leach into the food, especially if contents are high in fat.)

CHAPTER TAKEAWAY

Today, much innovation in food processing focuses on manipulating carbohydrates because they are inexpensive, versatile, and irresistible. We need carbs, but not the readily available Frankenfood imposters that our food system proliferates. The food industry may not have intended to take us away from more natural foods, but, over time, their focus has been on specific issues, such as pest control, crop yields, the rising cost of raw materials, refrigeration, distances between food sources and markets, growing regulations, changing consumer demand, and profits. Focus on these issues has come at the cost of healthy, fresh, nutritious food.

CHAPTER 2

THE STORY OF THE LOWLY SWEET POTATO

THE RISE, FALL, AND PROMISE OF THIS HUMBLE ROOT

A Beneficial Carb for Our Bodies in the Modern World

To thrive in this new world, our bodies need good, natural carbs that we were designed to eat. We need carbs that fill our muscles with energy and not our waistline with fat. We need carbs that release energy slowly and steadily. We need carbs that supply our body with nutrients. We need natural foods that are easy for our body to digest, replenishing our nutrient stores instead of depleting them. In addition, these good carbs need to compete against tempting Frankenfoods (bad carbs) not only in taste but also convenience.

Lucky for us, nature has made the sweet potato. Full of nutrition and energy, the sweet potato is a food that not only bolsters our health but can also compete in both taste and convenience with the bad carbs so plentiful in our modern world.

The Nutritional All-Star

The sweet potato is one of the world's power-packed, nutritionally-dense, super foods. But because of its name, it suffers the stigma of being both sweet (understood as sugar) and a potato (unhealthy). Despite its misleading name, the sweet potato is a nutritional all-star.

HERE ARE A FEW SWEET POTATO FACTS AND BENEFITS:

SWEET POTATOES HAVE MORE THAN 100 PERCENT OF THE DAILY REQUIREMENT FOR VITAMIN A (BETA-CAROTENE). They contain more vitamin A than any other fruit or vegetable. Vitamin A keeps our eyes in tip-top shape, helping our vision discriminate colors and handle low lighting. It also plays an important part in the body's defense against unstable chemical agents that can cause damage to the cells.

SWEET POTATOES CONTAIN HIGH AMOUNTS OF VITAMIN-E, AN ANTIODXIDANT THAT HELPS PROTECT OUR BODIES FROM FREE RADICALS. When passing through the digestive tract, sweet potatoes lower the potential health risks posed by heavy metals and oxidized free radicals.

SWEET POTATOES HAVE MORE FIBER PER SERVING THAN OATMEAL. More fiber provides a feeling of fullness and helps control food intake.

SWEET POTATOES ARE THE BEST SOURCE FOR BIOAVAILABLE (ABSORBABLE) BETA-CAROTENE; preferred over the much-touted dark, leafy green veggies. Thus, the body can absorb more of the plant's nutrients.

DESPITE BEING NATURALLY SWEET, SWEET POTATOES ARE A COMPLEX CARBOHYDRATE. Unlike white potatoes, they digest slowly and will not spike blood sugar.

SWEET POTATOES CONTAIN A NATURAL PROTEIN THAT HELPS REPAIR ITSELF WHEN DAMAGED. When digested, this protein is utilized as an anti-inflammatory in our bodies and helps repair cells.

THE CENTER FOR SCIENCE IN PUBLIC INTEREST (CSPI) HAS RANKED THE SWEET POTATO NUMBER ONE IN NUTRITION, more than 100 points ahead of spinach or broccoli.

THE PIÈCE DE RESISTANCE—SWEET POTATOES TASTE LIKE CAKE, so much goodness in an easily transportable package.

THE AMERICAS GIFT TO THE WORLD

When the Spanish explorers sailed to the Americas to find gold, they found treasure of another kind—the sweet potato. The indigenous peoples of South and Central America and Mexico had been extensively growing the sweet potato going back at least to 8,000BC. The "batata," or sweet potato, was a staple in their diets.

Christopher Columbus is credited with introducing the sweet potato to Europe. On his fourth voyage from the Caribbean, he presented the "batata" to Queen Isabella of Spain. The sweet potato became a highly prized gift and delicacy among the nobility. "A batata well-cured and well-prepared is just like fine marzipan," wrote a historian of the times. Another contemporary wrote that after curing and roasting, "they will taste as if they had been dipped in a jar of jam, they will be so honey-sweet." From Spain, the sweet potato traveled to Germany, Belgium, and England. Although cultivation was successful in Spain, the attempts to grow them in Northern Europe were only partly successful, as the sweet potato was better suited to the heat of a tropical climate.

The Golden Age of exploration carried the sweet potato eastward by Portuguese explorers to regions of Africa, India, Southeast Asia, and Indonesia. Spanish explorers brought sweet potatoes westward to Guam, the Philippines, and the East Indies. From the Philippines it traveled to China and from China to Japan. By the mid-sixteenth century the sweet potato was growing in most of the tropical areas with plentiful water around the world.

It is a mystery how the sweet potato spread to Polynesia. Long before the Spanish explorers discovered the sweet potato in the Americas, it was playing a role in the diet of the peoples of the South Pacific, New Zealand, Easter Island, and Hawaii. Most scholars believe that the ancient Polynesians voyaged to Peru, where they obtained sweet potatoes and, upon returning, planted them and dispersed them to other islands.

BATATA + PAPA = PATATA

The newly embraced sweet potato posed a name challenge to its appreciative European audience. The Spanish took the indigenous Taino name for the sweet potato, batata, directly, but they also later combined it with the Quechua (Inca) word for potato, papa, to create the word patata for the common potato, which arrived fifty to a hundred years later from the Americas. This provided considerable confusion between the sweet potato and the potato. Accounts show that the English frequently used sweet potato and potato interchangeably when they were first becoming acquainted with the new vegetables. Eventually, the sweet potato developed its own distinct identity. While the potato suffered a shady reputation during its early days of introduction in Europe, the sweet potato was prized for its sweetness and sought after by kings and nobles as a delicacy.

The Sweet Potato in Ole England

England's herbalist John Gerard wrote about the sweet potato in his 1597 Herball or Generall Historie of Plantes. He stated that the sweet potato "comforts, strengthens and nourishes the body," and also had the property of "procuring bodily lust." This aphrodisiac quality could be the reason for its popularity in the upper classes of sixteenth-century England.

It is suggested that Henry VIII consumed huge amounts of sweet potatoes, especially sweet potato pie. Shakespeare's Falstaff exclaims in the Merry Wives of Windsor (1602) "Let the sky rain potatoes (sweet). Let it thunder to the tune of 'Greensleeves,' hail kissing-comfits and snow eringoes!"

The Sweet Potato in Colonial America

The early colonists of Virginia were growing sweet potatoes by 1648, possibly earlier. The sweet potato was brought to them by explorers and traders from the West Indies and Mexico. Besides being tasty, it grew with relative ease and speed and in abundance. As the colonies expanded, the sweet potato became an item of trade to the northern colonies. The name "sweet potato" came into use after the 1740s as a means for the colonists to distinguish it from the white potato, which had been brought to New England by Scottish-Irish immigrants.

When things got tough during times of war and supplies of wheat and corn were limited, people turned to the sweet potato to carry them through. Weekly sweet potato rations were given to soldiers. Sweet potatoes were even made into a coffee substitute. During the Revolutionary War,

General Francis Marion, the "Swamp Fox" of South Carolina, maintained his men for months at a time on little else.

The Sweet Potato Comes to the Rescue of Many Nations

Beyond America's shore, the sweet potato has also been a valuable crop in times of food scarcity, even saving populations from starvation and famine. In 1593 facing a food shortage in their homeland, Chinese explorers found sweet potatoes growing on the island of Luzon. They recognized the value of sweet potatoes and brought them back to China. The sweet potato was quickly adopted, as it produced three to four times the quantity of food as rice planted on the same amount of land. Over the years, the sweet potato is credited with sustaining the Chinese population through numerous droughts that devastated native grain staples. China is now the world's largest producer of sweet potatoes.

In Japan the sweet potato was also prized as a famine-relief crop. Most recently the sweet potato was called upon to alleviate food shortages during World War II. After the war, its popularity declined in part due to its association with hardship.

Indonesian culture once relied heavily on the sweet potato, which grew plentifully in the local climate. When rice began to surpass it as a staple for breakfast, lunch, and dinner, the transition came at a cost to the population's health, as the poor suffered from malnutrition. Recently, fluctuations in world rice prices combined with population growth have made rice too expensive for many Indonesians. Once again, sweet potatoes are coming to the rescue. The government is making an effort to reintroduce the sweet potato as a staple, which will reduce malnutrition and help insulate citizens against fluctuating rice prices.

During the trying times of the Revolutionary and Civil Wars soldiers would boil the skin of sweet potatoes to make a substitute coffee.

In Uganda, the sweet potato came to the rescue in the 1990s when a virus ravaged cassava crops. Today in Sub-Saharan Africa, the sweet potato is outpacing the growth of other staples due to its high nutritional value, especially as a source of vitamin A.

The Spread of a New Diet: How the Sweet Potato Fell out of Favor

Foods have always been used as status symbols. What we eat broadcasts our knowledge, cultural alliances, and position in society. Up until the mid-twentieth century, the sweet potato ranked second only to the potato among vegetable crops in the United States. Unfortunately, despite its nutrition and reliability, the sweet potato again became associated with hard times. When people became more affluent, their diets changed and the sweet potato became less prominent as a food source.

This diet transition has happened around the world. Today in China the sweet potato serves as a vital component of country life, feeding both people and livestock with a nutritious, low-maintenance crop. While sweet potatoes have helped small farms thrive, industrial agriculture in China does not put as many resources toward the sweet potato as other crops. Technologies that could make sweet potato production more efficient have not been developed. As a result, Chinese farmers are beginning to grow more popular and profitable commodities, such as wheat and corn, which have better terms of trade than sweet potatoes. The end result is that fewer sweet potatoes are being grown. Once again, despite its nutritional advantage, the sweet potato is being underutilized.

The Health Promise of the Sweet Potato

The American diet, with a foundation of grains and refined sugar, has spread worldwide. With its widening reach, the health problems of modern civilization—obesity, diabetes, cardiovascular disease, etcetera also spread across the globe. We no longer face starvation in today's developed world. Instead we face a crisis of health caused by the foods—in particular the bad carbs—we eat. Lucky for us, we have the sweet potato. Increased consumption of the sweet potato in place of grains can help us combat many of the health issues damaging our nation and world.

The Sweet Potato's Place of Prominence in Okinawa

While in some cultures the sweet potato is the underdog, in other cultures the sweet potato is revered. Okinawans love the sweet potato. Noguni Soukan was a bureaucrat who brought the sweet potato to Okinawa from China in 1605. He planted seeds in his hometown, and because it was delicious, easy to cultivate, and nutritious, the magical food spread throughout the island.

In the streets of Okinawa today, you hear cart vendors yell at the top of their lungs "Yaki-Yaki-Yakimo." This is the call for oven-roasted goodness—the gooey, delicious sweet potato, caramelized to perfection and brought straight to your door. That's right, not ice cream: sweet potatoes. Sweet potatoes have become entrenched in Okinawa's diet and culture. One can find them everywhere—at the impulse-buy section in 7/11 stores, incorporated into Kit-Kat bars in the candy section, and at sacred temples to purchase as homage to past ancestors.

Every year thousands of people attend a sweet potato festival in Okinawa where they pay tribute to this super food. At the festival the community celebrates the harvest with music, beer, sweet potatoes, and sumo wrestling. Like American children hunting through gardens for Easter eggs, the children of Okinawa dig through mounds of dirt to find sweet potatoes. Taught to respect this honored root, kids read books devoted to the sweet potato and draw pictures of sweet potatoes dressed as super heroes. And, of course, when the time comes to request a treat, they ask for a sweet potato.

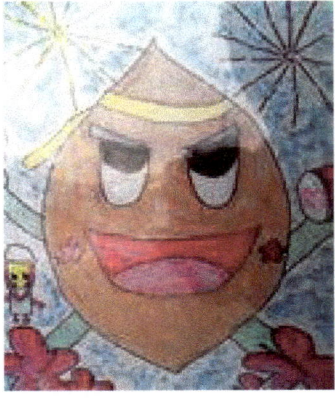

The Okinawan Way

Okinawans have the longest life expectancy in the world: 81.2 years compared with 76.8 in the United States. They not only live longer, they live healthier with lower levels of heart disease (80 percent less than in America) and almost no cancer or obesity. More Okinawans live into their hundreds than in any other culture.

How do they do it? Okinawans eat at least seven servings of vegetables daily. Sweet potatoes, bean sprouts, onions, and green peppers are prominent in their diet and fuel them to a long, healthy life.

The Sweet Potato versus the Potato

The sweet potato and potato are not related, not even distant cousins, even though both are indigenous to the Americas. The sweet potato (Ipomoea batatas) is a root from the morning glory family that grows best in temperate or tropical climates. The potato (Solanum tuerosum) is a tuber from the nightshade family and can grow in cooler climates and difficult terrains.

Both the sweet potato and potato are full of nutrition (the potato's poor health rap in recent years is due to the fact that over 75 percent of U.S. potato production goes into processed and fried products). Based on several key differences, however, reaching for a sweet potato is the smarter choice:

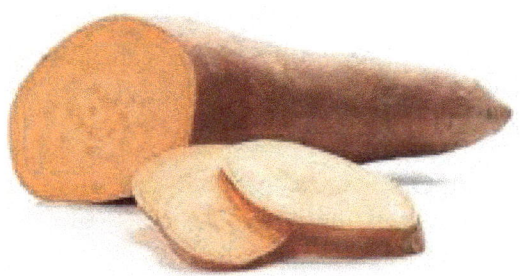

THE INCAS WORSHIPPED BOTH THE SWEET AND WHITE POTATO. ONE OF THEIR PRAYERS:

"O Creator! Thou who givest life to all things and hast made men that they may live, and multiply, multiply also the fruits of the earth, the potatoes and other food that thou hast made, that men may not suffer from hunger and misery."

A Comparison of Nutrition Between The Sweet Potato and The Potato

GLYCEMIC INDEX

....

SWEET POTATO LOW
WHITE POTATO HIGH

The sweet potato is a complex carbohydrate that is digested more slowly than a white potato and, therefore, will not cause blood sugar to spike. Slow digestion equals better management of energy, a benefit for your health.

DIETARY FIBER

....

SWEET POTATO 6.6 GRAMS

WHITE POTATO 4.2 GRAMS

Soluble fiber lowers bad LDL cholesterol by 1 percent for every 1–2 grams consumed daily. Because of its structure, the human gastrointestinal tract cannot digest soluble fiber, so as it passes through the system it helps with regularity.

BETA-CAROTENE (VITAMIN-A)

....

SWEET POTATO 400% THE DAILY VALUE

WHITE POTATO 0% THE DAILY VALUE

Sweet potatoes with bright, orange-colored flesh have four times the U.S. Recommended Daily Allowance for beta-carotene.

VITAMIN-C

....

SWEET POTATO 39.2 MG

WHITE POTATO 25.2 MG

Sweet potatoes provide more than half the daily requirement of vitamin C, an antioxidant that promotes cellular health and helps form collagen production.

ANTI-INFLAMMATORY

....

SWEET POTATO STRONGLY ANTI-INFLAMMATORY

WHITE POTATO MODERATELY INFLAMMATORY

While potatoes cause moderate levels of inflammation, sweet potatoes fight it. Eating anti-inflammatory foods gives our bodies the tools to help fight infections and heal.

Why Yams Are Really Sweet Potatoes and How Marketers Led Us Astray

Mention sweet potatoes and people wonder, what is the difference between a sweet potato and a yam? This baffling question has stumped many sweet potato lovers as they walk the produce aisle.

It will surprise most to know that "yams" in the United States and Canada are actually a variety of sweet potato. Most Americans have not seen a true yam. When an orange-fleshed variety of the sweet potato was introduced in the marketplace in 1937, the producers and marketers in the American South wanted to call it something different to distinguish it from the white-fleshed sweet potato that most people were used to. They called it a yam.

The word yam comes from the African word nyami. African slaves in the South called the sweet potato "nyami" because it reminded them of a starchy, edible tuber of that name that grew in their homeland. And so, the confusion began. Yams in the United States are actually sweet potatoes. Real yams are an entirely different plant altogether.

Sweet potatoes come in a variety of flesh colors that range from white to beige to orange to deep purple. Although the terms yam and sweet potato are generally used interchangeably in the United States, the Department of Agriculture requires that the label "yam" always be accompanied by "sweet potato."

True yams, as opposed to the yams that are labeled as such in U.S. supermarkets, are a starchy, edible tuber. It has a rough and scaly outside and a different nutritional makeup. Yams are cultivated for consumption primarily in Africa, Asia, and Oceania.

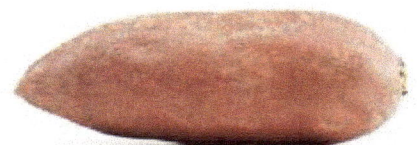
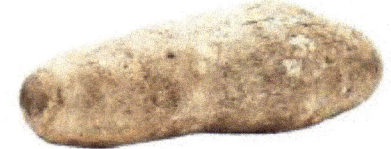

	Sweet Potato	**True Yam**
Plant Family	Morning Glory	Yam
Origin	Tropical zones Americas	Africa Asia
Edible portion of plant	Storage root	Tuber
Appearance	Smooth skin	Rough, scaly skin
Mouth Feel	Moist	Dry
Taste	Sweet	Starchy
Beta-Carotene	High	Very Low
Climate for growing	Tropical and temperate	Tropical
Availability	Grown in U.S.	Imported

SHAKESPEARE REFERS TO THE APHRODISIAC QUALITIES OF SWEET POTATOES IN THE MERRY WIVES OF WINDSOR.

"Let the sky rain sweet potatoes; let it thunder to the tune of 'Green Sleeves'; hail kissing-comfits and snow eringoes; let there come a tempest of provocation, I shelter me here."

CHAPTER TAKEAWAY

Our bodies are designed to thrive on nature's food, not food imposters. Technology has stripped many foods of their inherent nutrients, enhanced them with artificial additives, and created fake foods that crowd grocery shelves. While wheat, corn, and rice—recent diet additions in the long history of Homo sapiens—have become the popular carbohydrates of choice, the humble sweet potato is the one packed with nutrients that will keep our bodies healthy and waistlines slim. In the past when nations have faced famine and drought, the sweet potato has been the nutritious savior. While most do not experience starvation from lack of food, the Western diet does induce a nutritional starvation that results in poor health and disease. Full of the kind of nutrition and goodness that the human body has evolved to thrive upon, the sweet potato deserves a larger role in today's diet and a superstar spot on the table.

Part II

STOP SURVIVING, START THRIVING

A NEW EQUATION FOR OPTIMAL HEALTH

CHAPTER 3

CALORIES ARE NOT CREATED EQUAL

—

WHY FATS WON't MAKE YOU FAT, BAD CARBS ARE HEALTH CULPRITS, AND FRUCTOSE GIVES YOU THE LIVER OF AN ALCOHOLIC

From Trains to Grains: The Dubious Origins of the Calorie

Ask dieters what the key to weight loss is and they will tell you to burn more calories than you eat. In the mind of many, this idea has become so deified that it is now the single tool used for dieting. A product's calorie count has become so important that it has even migrated to the front label on some packaged goods. Even indulgent foods like cookies, juice, and alcohol boast low calories. Low-calorie has become synonymous with healthy. Where did this ubiquitous unit of measure come from? And how much does it actually tell us?

The calorie was a measurement invented during the Industrial Revolution. It was first conceived in the early nineteenth century by French physicist and chemist Nicolas Clément, who, among many other pursuits, studied the thermodynamics of steam in relation to powering steam engines. He came up with the notion of the calorie to provide a metric to accurately describe the potential energy of fuel. The calorie was defined as the quantity of heat needed to raise the temperature of 1 kilogram of water by 1 degree Celsius. For Clément's purposes, this rise in temperature transformed water to steam, and steam moved trains. Understanding how much heat was needed to produce steam was an important metric that helped differentiate between types of fuel.

A few decades later, a nutritionist named Wilbur Olin Atwater was seeking to understand the potential energy in food. His thought was that since "bodies are machines" and food is the fuel that runs those machines, he could apply Clément's notion of potential energy to food. Instead of incinerating coal or wood, he incinerated foods, such as mutton, rye bread, and pickled herring in a calorimeter. Different foods produced varying levels of heat. He reasoned that each food had a different energy potential, some burned fast and hot, and others burned slow and steady. With this information, he created a table giving popular foods each a caloric value. The notion of calories caught on.

If our bellies were incinerators and powered our bodies with combustion, calories would be a useful metric for us. However, our systems are more complex than steam engines. There's more to food than the heat it gives off. A calorie determined by how fast and hot a food burns is too simplistic a metric on which to base our discussion of nutrition.

A calorie is easy to understand and an appealing metric unit. It can be expressed by a number that represents the potential energy in a food, a simple concept to grasp. And this simplicity explains why calories have become the focal point for conversations about diet and nutrition. Unfortunately, our bodies are more complex. The calorie does not measure or make any differentiation in the way our bodies process different foods. If we want to move the conversation beyond oversimplified nutritional concepts, we have to understand more about how our bodies work—how we break down food and what happens afterward. Though this might get a little scientific, when armed with more knowledge we can better understand what our bodies ask of us and respond appropriately.

If our bellies were incinerators and powered our bodies with combustion, calories would be a useful metric.

Optimal Health is More Than Counting Calories

The calorie argument claims that, based on weight, age, and several other variables, we each need a specific number of calories per day. To lose, gain, or maintain weight in this model, you have two variables: calories consumed and calories expended.

According to this theory, to lose weight we simply eat less and move more. To gain weight, we move less and eat more. If we followed this simplified formula, we could eat Twinkies all day and run those calories off on a treadmill. However, common sense tells us this is not health. Sure, counting calories can help some people move in the right direction by eliminating the most egregious diet offenders, but for those who are serious about being healthy, simply counting calories doesn't make the cut. Counting calories does not help manage appetite or eliminate cravings, and these can be serious impediments to weight loss. It also doesn't help manage or reverse diseases. We need a more holistic model.

Weight loss is often one of the biggest single motivators for dietary changes, but optimizing our health offers a full slate of other benefits. When we are thriving, we are lean, strong, and full of energy. We are emotionally steady. We even have clearer skin. As a considerable added bonus, seeking optimal health today will have big payoff as we grow older.

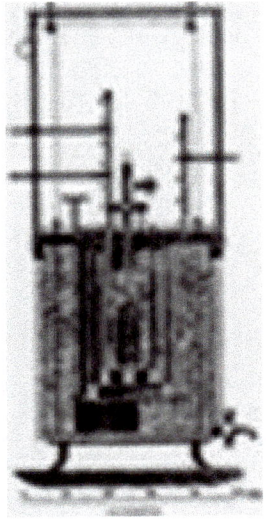

THE CALORIMETER USED FOR ATWATER'S EXPERIMENTS.

How the device worked: inside is a small cylinder in which the substance to be tested is burned, being mixed for this purpose with materials that furnish oxygen. The smaller cylinder is encased within a larger cylinder that holds water. The heat from the burning substance is transferred to the water and measured by the rise in temperature as shown by a thermometer.

IF OPTIMAL HEALTH IS WHAT YOU SEEK, HERE ARE FOUR PILLARS TO KEEP IN MIND

The Four Pillars Of Optimal Health: Food, Hormones, Low Inflammation, And Activity

When we start looking closely at our bodies, the science can get complicated fast. Don't be afraid. We only need to know the most basic concepts of each pillar in order to reap most of the benefits.

When thinking about the food pillar, we need to know how our bodies deal with the major macronutrients, specifically carbohydrates. For hormones we need to understand how our diet affects fat storage through the hormone insulin and the stress hormone cortisol. For inflammation we need to understand how the food we eat affects chronic inflammation. Finally, we need to look at our physical activity and see how it can be maximized to bolster our health.

These pillars can be the foundation for optimal health if you think about them in combination, making the concept of the four pillars a bit more sophisticated than a simple calculation of calories in and calories out. While food choice plays the largest role, your choices will be better informed if you also think about how the foods you choose affect hormones, inflammation, and ability to participate in physical activities. By making the right changes to what we eat, we will positively affect every system in our body.

Many people feel that food science, which helps us understand the body, is too complicated. However, a basic understanding of the four pillars can be rewarding.

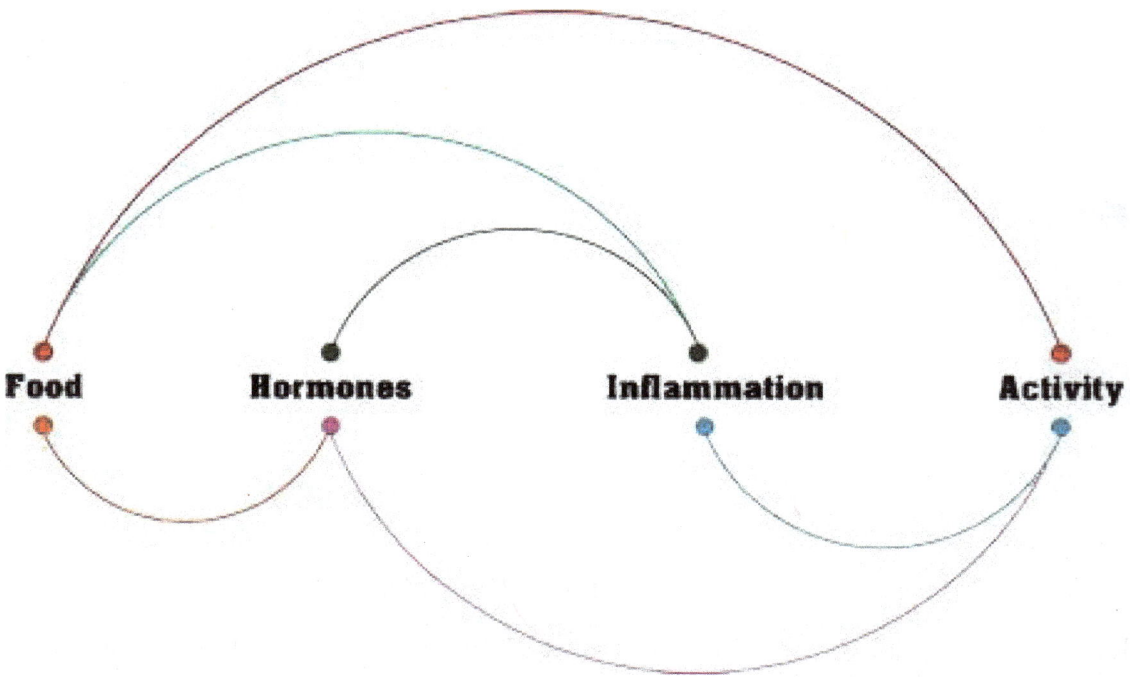

Food ⟷ Activities

Eating the right foods makes us energetic and compels us to be active. Eating the wrong foods leaves us lethargic and feeling depleted.

Food ⟷ Hormones

Eating large amounts of carbohydrates triggers the release of a hormone called insulin. One of insulin's roles is to send a signal to cells that they should absorb glucose from the blood stream. When carbohydrates are broken down into sugar (glucose), insulin helps shuttle excess glucose into the cells. Muscles and the liver fill up first. When they run out of room and blood glucose is still high, insulin shuttles that extra energy to be stored as fat.

Food ⟷ Inflammation

Eating the wrong foods wreaks havoc on the gut, weakening its defense against bad particles (undigested food/bacteria/other alien substances) that want to get into the bloodstream. When the invaders make it into the blood, the body fights back with an immune response, which triggers inflammation.

Inflammation ⟷ Hormones

Increased inflammation makes the body more resistant to the hormone insulin. When the body becomes insulin resistant, this hormone becomes less effective in doing its job. This means more insulin is needed to do the same amount of work. The pancreas (insulin factory) tires out.

Activity ⟷ Hormones

Activity elicits the right hormonal cocktail, stimulating the body to rebuild and strengthen. At the other extreme, overtraining puts excessive stress on the endocrine system (hormone factories). It gets rundown, overworked, and unable to effectively do its job (adrenal fatigue).

Activity ⟷ Inflammation

Strenuous activity breaks down muscle tissue, causing inflammation. When athletes engage in constant rigorous exercise, they can suffer from invisible chronic inflammation inside the body and in the bloodstream.

How the Body Turns Food into Fuel: The Disassembly Line of Digestion

Food supplies the raw material for our bodies' basic functions: growth and repair. When we eat, our bodies begin to disassemble food into usable nutrients, including the three macronutrients: carbohydrates, proteins, and fats. These nutrients play different but essential roles.

Carbohydrates serve our cells as fast-acting fuel. When they enter our system, they are broken down into simple sugars, including glucose, lactose, and fructose. Our bodies utilize these sugars differently: glucose is sent directly into the bloodstream to feed activity, repair, and the replication of cells; lactose is digested into even smaller sugars—galactose and glucose; and fructose is sent to the liver to be processed and stored.

Glucose is the most common of these simple sugars. It fuels our muscles and our metabolism. Most importantly, glucose fuels our brain. The brain needs the most glucose and requires a steady stream to keep up with its to-do list of functions.

Carbohydrates and their sugars are processed at varying speeds. Complex carbohydrates, which make up vegetables, such as broccoli, kale, and sweet potatoes, are full of fiber, so they take longer for the body to break down. Complex carbohydrates slow down the rate at which foods move through the stomach (gastric emptying) and determine the speed of nutrient absorption. Simple carbohydrates, such as sugar, sweet beverages, and candy, enter our blood stream quickly, providing a jolt of energy in the form of a glucose surge. Fruit and packaged foods contain a significant amount of fructose, which goes straight to the liver (where much of it is turned into fat) instead of to hungry cells. We will explore the different journeys of glucose and fructose and how those journeys have consequences for our health.

Glucose (sugar) is the energy that powers our cells. At times we have more glucose circulating in our system than necessary for immediate use. The body prudently wants to store glucose for later and sends it to one of three storage banks. The muscles act as the first storage bank, storing glucose to fuel bursts of intense activity. This is energy that is conveniently stored and easy to access. Since muscles lack the enzyme that exports glucose from cells, the glucose in muscles is destined to fuel activity. While storing glucose in muscle cells is desirable, storage space is finite. Excess glucose that can no longer fit in the muscles has a different fate.

Excess glucose is sent to the liver for storage. The liver is a flexible energy bank that can deal with deposits (excess glucose in the system) and withdrawals (sending glucose into the system when glucose is low). Energy stored in the liver is easy to access and steadies the body's glucose levels between meals or during sleep. As with the muscles, the liver has a finite storage capacity. When it is full, excess energy is sent into long-term storage.

FAT IS THE BODY'S LONG-TERM SAVINGS ACCOUNT. THE BODY DOES NOT EASILY GIVE UP THESE "HARD-EARNED" STORES.

Fat or adipose tissue is the body's long-term savings account and the third storage bank. We are born with a given number of fat cells, which expand and contract based on how much extra energy they are storing. When the body has enough energy in the muscles and the liver, the excess makes its way into long-term storage, meaning the fat cells. This fat savings is kept as insurance against scarcity in the future and is harder for the body to access compared to energy in the muscles and liver. The body does not easily give up these "hard-earned" stores. It only takes the trouble of releasing this energy when dietary levels of glucose in the rest of the body are low or during extended moderate metabolic activities.

Carbs are not the only source of glucose. The body can also derive glucose from fats and proteins. However, since the process of turning these other macronutrients into glucose takes more time, our body directs us to eat carbs when we crave energy. Like an addict that knows how to get a quick fix, our body knows what will get into the bloodstream fastest. Carbs! As with other substances that give us the most immediate boost, they are addictive.

Protein, derived from the Greek word for "of prime importance," is the fundamental building material for the body. Protein is required for the operation of every cell's metabolic activity. It is the second most common molecule in the body after water. The brain, bones, skin, muscles, blood, hair, and connective tissue are all made up primarily of protein. Protein also forms the antibodies we create to fight off disease, as well as some hormones that regulate our body's activity.

When we eat protein, our body breaks it down into its basic building blocks—amino acids. These amino acids can then be reassembled into the various proteins necessary for the body's essential activities, such as construction of bones, muscles, cartilage, skin, and blood. These amino acids are also used to make enzymes and hormones. As soon as protein enters the digestive system, it begins to be broken down and put to work. Unlike carbohydrates or fats, protein is not stored.

Twenty different amino acids are incorporated into various peptides and proteins. Our bodies can manufacture some, but nine of those amino acids only come from food plants, poultry, meat, fish, nuts, and eggs.

When carbohydrate intake is limited and blood glucose is low, the body utilizes glucogenic amino acid (found in protein) to make glucose. The process, gluconeogenesis, is slow but provides a stable, though limited, source of glucose.

When we eat protein, hormones released in our stomach and gut make us feel full and satiated. These "I'm full" hormones (cholecystokinin, peptide YY, ghrelin, and insulin) signal the body to stop eating.

Fats are essential to the human body. They are broken down into fatty acids that help form cell membranes and hormones. They are also stored throughout the body and are available for use as an energy source or to regulate body temperature and cushion the organs.

THE BODY WILL NOT GO TO THE TROUBLE OF DIPPING INTO FAT STORES UNLESS GLUCOSE IN THE DIET IS LOW.

In times of need, the liver can convert fats into glucose, our body's go-go juice. For the body to make one glucose molecule, two triglyceride (fat) molecules are required. The process is inefficient and demands extra resources. As a result, the body will not go through the trouble of synthesizing glucose from fats unless sugars are low.

Like protein, fats trigger the release of "I'm full hormones" (cholecystokinin, peptide YY, ghrelin, and insulin). Since fats take a long time to break down in the digestive system, this feeling of fullness lasts longer.

With a carb-restricted diet, your body can run off its own storage supply—the excess fat on your tush and belly. In general when you eat more calories from fat and protein than from carbs, your body begins the transition to burning its own fat. This transition takes some time, as your body adjusts to processing the new form of fuel (fat). Once your system has shifted from carbs to fat as the primary source of fuel, you are said to be "fat-adapted." That's a good thing!

When carbs are severely limited in a diet, a person enters into ketosis, a state of intense fat burning. This diet is getting more and more attention, as it has been used by doctors in battling cancer, eliminating epileptic seizures, and preventing the progression of degenerative brain diseases, such as Alzheimer's. To learn more about ketosis, check out the quick-start guide in the self-monitoring section.

TIPS FOR MANAGING YOUR CRAVINGS:

Your body asks, sometimes shouts, for what it needs. These cravings can be so loud they are impossible to ignore. The trick is to manage these messages so they don't derail your diet. Resisting food is not about will power—it's about interpreting the body's message correctly. To do this we need to understand the reason behind the body's request.

BE SURE YOU ARE HUNGRY Before eating, take a moment to listen to your body. Are you eating because you are bored? Do you need a break? Are you perpetuating a bad habit? If the answer is yes to any one of these, change your space. Go for a walk or go sit in a different spot.

This change in physical space can shift your mental space and provide the extra stimulation needed to shrug off a bad habit. If you feel you are genuinely hungry, eat smartly.

DRINK A GLASS OF WATER BEFORE YOU EAT What we call hunger is often thirst that's misinterpreted. Before sitting down to an irregularly scheduled meal or snack, drink a glass of water. Wait for half an hour and check in with your body again.

EAT FOODS YOUR BODY NEEDS, NOT WHAT IT ASKS FOR If your blood sugar is low, your body will ask for the foods to provide the quickest energy. This craving is often for sweets or other fast-acting fuels. Eat protein or fat to meet your body's short-term needs and even out long-term energy. A handful of nuts, a spoonful of almond butter, a piece of chicken, or a couple of slices of deli meats will serve you better and get you off the energy roller coaster. Properly fed, your body will stop craving sugar. Willpower no longer has to be the factor that determines success.

DON'T DRINK SUGAR WATER When your body asks for soda or juice, your body pretends it is saying, "I am thirsty." But it is also saying "Why drink water, when I can have extra sugar to store up fat for the coming winter?" Unless you want to store lots of excess fat in your cells, choose water over juice. You can find your vitamins in healthier places.

EAT BEFORE YOU ARE DESPERATE Desperation is a powerful force to derail your diet. Don't get stuck without good fuel. Plan ahead. Store stashes of fats and protein in your desk, glove box, or bag, such as beef jerky, tuna packs, and single-serving nut butter packets.

EATING SWEET POTATOES WITH A BIT OF FAT ALLOWS FOR SLOWER dIGESTION AND MORE VITAMIN A UPTAKE INTO CELLS.

Why Some Foods Leave You Feeling Fatigued

As we eat, nutrients are not digested in the order in which they enter our bodies. Instead, they are prioritized according to how fast our bodies can break them down. Carbohydrates, the fastest to process into simple sugar fuel, are absorbed first. Proteins, which are broken down into component amino acids, are next. Finally, the body tackles fats.

Foods that burn slowly, such as fats and proteins, provide a consistent stream of energy, making you feel full and satisfied longer. Carbohydrates, on the other hand, are processed comparatively quickly, giving you spikes of sugar in the bloodstream.

Simple carbs are broken down quickly and create a KABAM! in your system. Like a junky on crack, sugars are mainlined in the body, giving the initial feelings of super-human energy, giddiness, and invincibility. However, this high quickly comes crashing down, often resulting in feelings of low energy or motivation and the need for naptime. Many of the nutritionally unaware eat their way out of this inevitable slump by ingesting more carbs, spiking blood sugar back up and continuing the yo-yo effect throughout the day. Little do they know, by turning to this so-called solution, the problem intensifies.

In the 1800's when many sawmills were buzzing, big logs would be cut down into planks for building. In the process of cutting those logs, various sizes of wood would result, ranging from large wood chunks to sawdust. Some of the wood dust was so fine, the particulate would just float in the air, filling up the sawmill. With this volatile, combustible air in a confined space, smoking at a job site was dangerous. Sometimes sparks or other flames caught the air on fire, causing huge explosions.

Carbohydrates are like the different sizes of wood in the sawmill. Complex carbohydrates are the larger chunks, which may take some time to get started, but provide excellent fuel and burn in a controlled way. Do you want to know what soda and juice do to your system? Simple carbohydrates are like the wood dust particulate in the air that can combust, exploding in your system, wreaking havoc, and making mischief.

Complex carbohydrates are much less ominous. With more elaborate sugar structures, the fiber in foods like sweet potatoes and other vegetables, such as broccoli, kale, and cauliflower slows down the glucose dump into your system. A steady stream of glucose, instead of a quick flood, allows your body to manage energy flows more efficiently and without the side effects of an energy crash later. Properly fueled in this way all afternoon, you can run circles around your friends and colleagues, while they sit in their post-lunch haze.

Carbohydrate Spectrum

Simple carbs enter the system quickly. Complex carbs take longer. Proteins and fat are absorbed most slowly. Given the same number of calories, the illustration below gives you an idea of the rates various types of carbohydrates enter into the body.

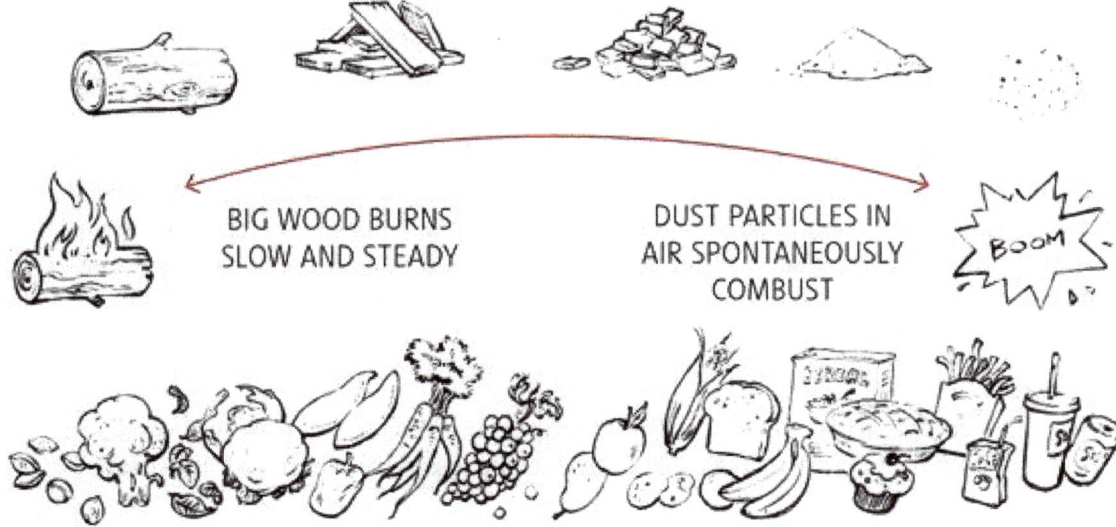

Ideal Glucose Chart

- Steady glucose means consistent energy throughout the day.
- Body feels alert, sharp, and has optimal energy without receiving cues to store more fat.

- Absence of low dips keeps ravenous hunger at bay.

Non-ideal
Glucose Chart

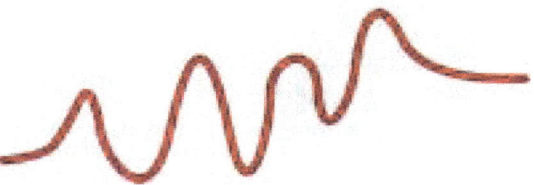

- Big swings in energy with pronounced highs and lows shortly after eating meals.
- Low periods characterized by lack of energy, sleepiness, mental fogginess, and hunger, even after eating.
- Low levels of glucose trigger the body to be hungrier more often.
- Coping mechanisms developed to deal with lows, include eating, caffeinating, sleeping, or even exercising.
- Spikes in glucose are hard for the body to manage. As stress piles upon stress, you develop "glucose creep," where glucose levels rise throughout the day.
- Consistently high blood sugar can lead to chronically elevated insulin in the body. The result? Your body never dips into fat stores and you pile on the weight without the chance to burn it off. Combined with leptin resistance (due to elevated triglycerides), high inflammation, and intestinal permeability, you have a recipe for obesity and autoimmune diseases.

Carb Monsters and the Danger of Over-Sugaring Your Kids

Kids are cute, except when they are not. Often bad parenting is not to blame. The culprit is bad feeding. Pint-sized people experience extreme swings of blood sugar on diets high in carb-rich foods, such as fruit juice, cereals, and bagels that cause momentary bursts of energy followed by crashes. If you were on a sugar-induced roller coaster, you would be yelling, screaming, and stomping your feet in public as well. Excessive sugar consumption influences everything, including mood, attention span, energy, and cognitive ability. For kids, this translates to tantrums, hyperactivity, attention deficit disorder, and poor performance in school.

Just like adults, kids need quality food. Even if they are less self-aware, their little bodies and brains react to the octane in their system. Set them up for success. Give them real nutrition.

How Orange Juice Became a Breakfast Staple

Orange juice became commercialized in 1910. Overproduction of citrus fruit that year meant that orchards were in danger of being cut down and crop prices were plummeting. Seeking to find new ways to market their surplus, orange growers applied the technology of pasteurization to kill bacteria that cause rot in orange juice. This extra processing made juice shelf-stable and shippable to cities around the country. Because of its lower price, pasteurized orange juice replaced the more traditional breakfast accompaniment of stewed fruit, thus stripping the traditional breakfast of its beneficial fiber while adding even more fructose to the mix.

TIPS FOR TEACHING KIDS GOOD EATING BEHAVIORS:

SAY NO TO JUICE
Feeding your child juice is like serving up a liquefied candy bar. If you must serve juice, dilute it generously with water. If flavor is what your kids are after, check out other non-juice options, such as Hint water, which infuses fruits without adding sugar or scary preservatives. Kids lived without juice for thousands of years. They can live without it now.

IF FOOD IS ENTERTAINMENT, CHOOSE YOUR TREATS WISELY
If keeping your babes occupied and quiet is the goal, try giving them goodies that won't spike their blood sugar. Make your own treats to store ahead of time and dole them out when you are ready for a little peace and quiet.

MAKE SNACK TIME INTO HEALTH FOOD TIME
Grab-and-go, prepackaged, convenience foods fill kids up with empty calories, make them overexcited, and leave them in a sugar-induced daze. Instead, serve vegetables when kids are hungry on the playground and in the sand box. Kids will learn to love what you give them. The sooner you get them going on nature's finest, the more they will love, crave, and ask for it.

ENERGY BARS ARE NOT FOR SMALL PEOPLE
Don't be a sucker for marketing. Energy bars are just socially permissible candy bars. If you want to feed your kid candy, own up to it, and feed them candy. Just because energy bars claim to be "good" for athletes doesn't mean they are good for kids.

MODEL GOOD BEHAVIOR
Monkey see, monkey do. Your kids will love what you love. Fill your plate with good foods from the ground, and they will learn to do the same. Unfortunately, lots of kids pick up unhealthy cues from television commercials and schoolmates. Be vigilant about being a good example.

PREPARE FOODS WITH YOUR KIDS
We all love what we make. It's no different for kids. Help them play a part in preparation and cooking. Chances are they will be more invested in eating their own nutritious concoctions.

STAY AWAY FROM THE KID'S MENU
Forty years ago, a kid's meal on the menu did not exist. Avoid at all costs the kaleidoscope of processed browns and tans: chicken nuggets, hot dogs, mac and cheese, fries, and so on. Feed your kids what you would eat. Smaller portions are good, but different foods are not. Color can be a helpful guide—fill your child's plate with the full range of colors found in nature's foods.

PACK YOUR KID'S LUNCH
No one is more invested in your family's health than you. School lunches are determined by prices and politics. Bad carbs win both battles. Keep your kids thriving by packing good, nutritious foods. Their better grades and teachers' good reports will make the extra effort worth it. Bad nutrition can result in crazy behavior, attention deficit disorder, and the start of a reliance on prescription medications for problems that could have been avoided with good food.

DON'T REWARD WITH FOOD
Our happy places are set early in life. When we grow up and life gets tough, we turn to those patterned behaviors to comfort us in bad times. Set the foundation for a good relationship with food from an early age by giving your children non-food rewards.

SUPERVISE SPORT SNACKS

Drinks and snacks that are marketed to athletes are high in carbs and sugar. They should not be on Little League refreshment tables. Just because your kids are running around on a playing field does not mean you should let them drink or eat sugar. Instead, find alternative beverages and snacks to keep your children fueled with the good stuff.

Managing Carbohydrates: Get Energy through Sweet Potato Power

Carbs are typically the foundation of every meal, but they are overrated compared to their macronutrient neighbors—protein and fat. While proteins and fats provide sustained energy, carbs in their common processed form just give us a boom and bust. Get off the roller coaster. Replace the fast carbs from sugars and grains in your diet with slow carbs from nature's vegetable bounty.

The sweet potato is a complex carbohydrate rich in potential energy. Full of fiber, it gradually releases its payload of fuel, rather than exploding like sawdust in the system for a quick energy high. When you incorporate sweet potatoes into meals and snacks, your cells get energy that burns long and steady.

WHAT YOU CAN DO ABOUT CARBS FOR OPTIMAL HEALTH:

REPLACE FAST-BURNING FOODS, such as wheat-based products (bread, pasta, or cereal) with slow-burning foods, such as vegetables and sweet potatoes.

MANAGE YOUR CRAVINGS SMARTLY by eating foods that will fuel your body needs (fat, protein, and slow-burning carbs), not what it asks for (sweets, sugar, and bad, simple carbs).

The Role of Sugar in our Evolutionary Biology

When we were hunters and gatherers long ago, seasons played a big role in our lives. How we adapted to availability of food during times of plenty affected how we survived when the pickings were scarce. Our systems evolved in a time when food was not abundant, and our bodies developed clever strategies to compensate. Response to sweetness was one of them.

As summer came into full bloom and trees were heavy with fruit, nature's bounties were plenty. For a short period of time, we had access to more food than we needed to meet our immediate survival needs. Our bodies learned to take advantage of the abundance in this short season to make preparations for winter. This meant taking excess sugar from fruit and storing it as fat. To do this we needed to eat, eat, and eat without getting full. Fructose, the sugar in fruit, bypassed the mechanism for fullness so that we could eat until the fruit was no longer available and plump up for the coming scarcity.

Our body's strategy for dealing with this once-seasonal sugar allowed us to pack away reserves for later in the form of fat. When winter came and nourishment was scarce, our bodies would dip into the fat storage for needed energy. The process of breaking down fat into fuel for the body results in glucose and a by-product called ketone bodies (a metabolic equivalent of glucose), fuel that keeps us going in times of scarcity. The problem today is that winter never comes. We no longer face those periods of scarcity that cued us to dip into our fat storage. We have also upped the amount of sugar in our diets. Thus, we store more and more fat without ever clearing out the storage bins.

FRUCTOSE, THE SUGAR IN FRUIT, BYPASSES OUR FULLNESS MECHANISM. LONG AGO, WE COULD EAT AND EAT TO STORE UP FOR WINTER. TODAY, WHILE FRUCTOSE IS ABUNDANT, WINTER NEVER COMES.

Not All Sugars are Created Equal

Our bodies break down carbohydrates into three types of simple sugar for processing—glucose, fructose, and galactose. Foods that are sweet to the taste have some combination of these molecules. For example, sucrose, common table sugar, is made up of one glucose molecule and one fructose molecule. The dairy sugar lactose, on the other hand, is made up of one galactose molecule and one glucose molecule.

These three different crystalline structures common in our food have different levels of sweetness to the taste. Fructose is the sweetest of all naturally occurring carbohydrates—sweeter than any other sugars, including common table sugar or honey. Glucose is the next sweetest, while galactose is much less sweet.

The sugars differ by more than just varying sweetness levels; their chemical make-ups have important health implications as well. Glucose and fructose have different chemical structures that affect the ways our bodies process and metabolize them.

Relative Sweetness of Sugars and Sweeteners

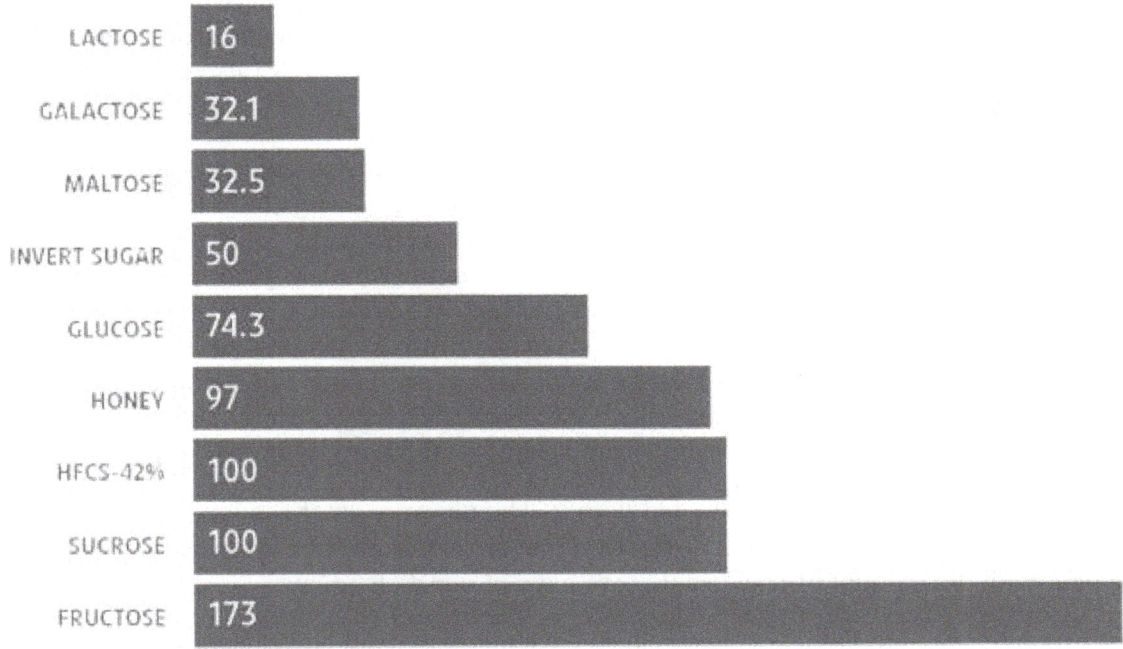

Numbers represent relative sweetness with table sugar (sucrose) defined as 100.

To understand their unique roles in our biology, let's follow their paths through the body. When we take a big bite of cake, it travels to the stomach where the cake is churned and broken apart by stomach acid. Once the cake has been mashed up into smaller particles, the remaining bits travel to the small intestine. When the sucrose or table sugar in the cake hits the intestinal wall, the molecules are broken into their two main components—glucose and fructose. Once separated, these molecules are off on their own paths.

GLUCOSE CAN BE USED BY EVERY CELL IN THE BODY. fRUCTOSE CAN ONLY BE METABOLIZED IN THE LIVER WHERE It IS LIKELY TURNED TO FAT.

Glucose goes directly into the bloodstream and can be utilized by any cell in the body. Our cells take that energy and use it to fuel our brains, to rebuild muscles, or to go about our daily lives.

In contrast to glucose, most fructose can only be metabolized by the liver, which has special enzymes to break it down. So instead of moving throughout the entire body, fructose must travel through the liver to be metabolized and turned into energy. As you can imagine, if we increase fructose in our diets, the liver will have lots of extra work.

Fructose: From Rare Treat to Ubiquitous Commodity

Long ago fructose was relatively scarce in the human diet. When fruit or other fructose-filled goodies became available, it was generally only for a short time, and we often had to compete with other sugar-loving animals to win our share of the spoils. Since this sugar was so valuable, the way the body processed this rare commodity was an asset for survival.

Today, fructose is in abundance. Fruits, once available for only a short season, are now ripe and ready to eat any day of the year. And, over the centuries, fruits have been selectively bred for higher sweetness levels—this means more fructose. Every day many Americans dress their morning breakfasts with these colorful sugar bombs and slurp liquid fructose (also known as juice), delivering a concentrated blast of fructose to the liver.

Fructose, beyond occurring naturally in fruit, has made its way into just about everything that is packaged in the form of high-fructose corn syrup (HFCS). HFCS is a particularly insidious form of sugar that is refined from corn instead of sugarcane or beets. Technically known by the food industry as HFCS-55 (a concoction composed of 55 percent fructose and 45 percent glucose), it was created to be indistinguishable to the palate from sucrose. In addition to good flavor and inexpensive production, HFCS allows packaged foods to stay fresh longer and gives a flaky texture to baked goods. Foods with HFCS are also less likely to crystallize when cooled, making them less susceptible to freezer burn. Sports drinks, breads, peanut butter, yogurt, canned vegetables, fruit juices, ice cream, sodas, candies, and cakes—all have a hefty amount of HFCS.

Fructose is everywhere. Our systems are loaded with it. The unaware eater can have fructose in every bite of every meal, leading to levels of fructose that are sky high. Our systems were not designed to deal with the amount of fructose that we have in our diets today.

The Gifts of Fructose: An Alcoholic's Liver, a Jacked Metabolism, and Never Feeling Full

As packaged food became more prevalent, fructose-rich sweeteners started to replace sucrose (table sugar). Fructose in the form of HFCS is not only sweeter and cheaper than sucrose, it was originally thought to have health benefits. Consumers and health experts originally loved the short-term effect fructose had on blood sugar. While glucose went straight into the bloodstream, fructose went to the liver, thus avoiding glucose spikes. But more than just avoiding glucose spikes, fructose in the absence of glucose reduced blood sugar. By simulating hepatic glucokinase, an enzyme that helps metabolism, the liver is turned into a glucose sponge and soaks up extra glucose in the blood stream. Everyone was happy: both sugar addicts and health experts finally agreed on an acceptable sugar. Fructose was instantly dubbed the healthier alternative. But the accolade had been bestowed too soon.

Fructose has its own drawback. It may not spike your glucose and insulin levels, but in large amounts it forces the liver into overdrive. When the liver is too full of fructose, the sugar turns into fat that stays in the liver, where there's little chance it can be turned into energy. If you ever want to burn that fat, your body first has to be running extremely low on glucose. Little chance of that happening on today's carb-heavy diet.

SUGAR IS A SOMETIMES DRUG AND SHOULD ONLY BE USED RECREATIONALLY.

Forty years ago fructose was deemed the most "lypogenic" carbohydrate—the carbohydrate that turns to fat most readily. Clever marketing, increased sweetness (as fruits are selectively bred and hybridized), prolonged shelf life, and year-round availability have helped us forget this fact.

The bad consequences of fructose go beyond its propensity to turn into fat. Fructose triggers a domino effect in our bodies that causes a change in metabolism. Under the influence of fructose, our muscles and fat become resistant to insulin, which in turn influences how nutrients are stored. The result? We get fatter.

The litany of detrimental side effects continues. Although packed with calories, fructose won't tell your brain that your body is full. The hypothalamus is the appetite control center in the brain—your internal nutrient counter. Hormones serve as messengers to tell the brain if the body is hungry or full. Depending on what hormones are circulating (insulin, leptin, cholecystokinin, and ghrelin), we are told when to eat, when to keep eating, and when to put down the fork. Fructose, however, does not stimulate any of these "enough to eat" hormones. This is why you can eat fruit all day long and never feel full.

Fructose is far from being the sugar savior it was once hailed as. It breeds fat in the liver, leaves you ravenously hungry, causes insulin resistance, and results in hyperinsulinemia (a condition where there is excess insulin compared to what is expected based on glucose levels). Elevated insulin directly inhibits the metabolism of stored fat. So, with fructose you eat more, get fat, and then stay fat because it's harder to dip into energy stores. It's a real lose-lose (or perhaps a weight gain-gain!) situation.

WHAT YOU CAN DO ABOUT SUGARS FOR OPTIMAL HEALTH:

ELIMINATE ALL PROCESSED FOODS WITH FRUCTOSE FROM YOUR DIET, including condiments and juice, also known as liquid fructose.

AVOID THE HABIT OF EATING FRUIT AS A DAILY SNACK just because it's convenient. Make batches of On-the-Go Sweet Potato Quiches, Sweet Potato Rainbow Cubes, and Sweet Potato Poppers from the recipe section, or make a simple steamed sweet potato to carry with you and munch on-the-go.

USE THE TASTINESS OF REAL FRUIT SPARINGLY to enhance dishes with flavor and variety.

WHEN YOU CRAVE SUGAR, TAKE ADVANTAGE OF THE SWEET POTATO for low fructose sweet satisfaction.

CHAPTER TAKEAWAY

Fructose is clearly a villain. Unless we are vigilant about spotting and eliminating hidden fructose in our foods, fructose weasels its way into our diets. It's hidden in fruit, table sugar, and, most insidious of all, high-fructose corn syrup. High fructose corn syrup in turn is found in products lining every shelf in the supermarket. Fructose is pervasive. Unlike glucose, the universal cell energy source, all this super-sweet fructose goes straight to your liver, where it has a high likelihood of turning into fat. To make matters worse, our brains don't know when to stop eating it.

How do we escape this nutritional nightmare? If you remove packaged foods from your diet, you have done much of the work cutting fructose out of the equation. If you want to eliminate even more, get to know the varying levels of fructose in fruits and vegetables. Sweet potatoes have less fructose than any other starchy vegetable, and their fructose levels are far lower than fruit. When you eat sweet potatoes, you get a healthy dose of good old glucose to fuel your body without the negative side effects of fructose.

CHAPTER 4

HORMONES: MANAGING THE BODY'S TRAFFIC SIGNALS

MAKING HORMONES WORK FOR YOU TO AVOID FAT STORAGE, MAXIMIZE SATISFACTION FROM FOOD, AND USE STRESS TO MAKE YOU STRONGER, NOT WEAKER

Hormones: The Body's Communication Network

Our bodies are made up of many different systems: circulatory, digestive, muscular, nervous, respiratory, reproductive, urinary, lymphatic, immune to name a few. While each system has a different function, they have to work together toward a common goal. To get on the same page, our bodies communicate with hormones. Hormones are chemical messengers sent throughout the blood to tell the rest of the body what's going on and how to behave.

When hormones are mentioned, most people immediately think of sex hormones: testosterone and estrogen . But while most people are familiar with these hormones, various other types of hormones circulate through our bodies at any given time, and their levels are affected by our environment. What we eat, how we sleep, how we work out, and our levels of stress all affect the messages our bodies are circulating. If we want to keep our bodies looking like Greek gods and goddesses, we need to make sure that our hormones are sending out the right marching orders. Not enough sleep, too much stress, or too little exercise can all have adverse effects on hormonal signaling and, ultimately, our waistlines.

Insulin: Hormone of Utmost Importance

The system of hormones in our bodies can seem complicated to the casual observer. But one hormone in particular is worth the extra effort in order to understand how the foods we eat affect our bodies: insulin.

When excess glucose is circulating through the bloodstream, insulin directs the glucose to one of the body's three storage banks—the muscles, the liver, or, if those two are full, the fat cells (adipose tissues). Insulin activates one of the keys (lipoprotein lipase) to open up fat cells' doors to store excess glucose, amino acids, and even lipids (fat) in the event of famine. When opened, the fat cells transform glucose to fat for long-term storage.

In sum insulin helps make us fat. High levels of insulin in our blood mean more glucose is shuttling into the adipose cells to be transferred into fat. Low levels of insulin mean fewer glucose-to-fat transformations. Unfortunately, the diet recommended by the USDA and other experts is high in carbohydrates, especially fructose, which results in insulin resistance coupled with high glucose levels in the blood. High glucose sends insulin soaring and waistlines bulging. If we control our insulin, we will feel terrific and be lean into our twilight years.

Insulin and Glucagon: The Tag Team Hormones That Keep Energy Flowing

Glucose is the cell's main energy source. Without it our cells are like cars without gas. They won't keep running. The pancreas detects levels of glucose in the blood to make sure that our cells are never running on empty, whether we are stuffed, starving, sleeping, or active. Responding to glucose levels, the pancreas produces two types of hormones—insulin and glucagon.

When glucose levels are high, the beta cells of the pancreas produce insulin. This hormone circulates in our blood directing the storage of glucose in cells—in muscle, liver, and fat cells. Insulin reduces the concentration of glucose in the bloodstream.

When blood glucose levels are low, such as between meals or when sleeping, alpha cells of the pancreas produce glucagon. This hormone directs the liver to transform glycogen (the long polysaccharide form of stored glucose) into glucose, which is then released into the blood. Glucose rises. Together, insulin and glucagon work to maintain a steady supply of glucose, that is, energy, to our cells and, most importantly, to the brain. These hormones send marching orders to our cells and tell them whether energy should be stored or released.

Insulin: Get the Concept or Get Fat

Back to carbohydrates. When we eat carbs, especially simple ones that explode quickly in our system, glucose is quickly released into our blood. As glucose levels rise, the pancreas receives a signal to secrete insulin. Insulin causes cells in the liver, muscles, and fat tissue to take up glucose from the blood and convert it into glycogen for storage. Think of glycogen as a cell's storage system for the body to easily access energy later.

Nature designed our bodies to work best with the natural foods in the environment of long ago. Nature's foods had a slow and steady release of energy at an unhurried pace. Today the foods we eat have excessive amounts of glucose that explode quickly in our blood. Coupled with high fructose levels and increased insulin resistance, more insulin is needed to do the same amount of work to control blood glucose. It is hard for the body to keep up with the demands on insulin production. Demands are so high that beta cells, the insulin factories of the pancreas, have to work in overdrive. With the rise in demand, the pancreas tries its best to increase supply. But under this kind of duress, over long periods of time, the beta cells of the pancreas get tired and can no longer keep up the pace. Exhausted, these overworked cells suffer from early cell death (apoptosis). Our pancreas no longer has the capabilities to produce the insulin necessary to control glucose levels. The inability of your pancreas to keep up with insulin production is one of the causes of type 2 diabetes.

When our pancreas gets fatigued, so do our cells. Hormones are like nagging parents: when they are constantly telling the cells to do the same thing over and over again, the cells simply tune them out (like rebellious children). When we have consistently high levels of insulin circulating through our system, our cells stop listening to their marching orders. In order to be heard, the insulin message has to get louder—requiring even more work of the already overworked pancreas. This vicious cycle is called insulin resistance. When we are insulin resistant, our cells need more insulin to do the same job. Gone unchecked, this is another cause that can lead to type 2 diabetes.

IN JAPAN THE SWEET POTATO HAS BEEN USED MEDICALLY TO TREAT DIABETES AND HELP INSULIN SENSITIVITY.

Still think this insulin warning does not apply to you? Let's try another angle: fat. High levels of insulin increase the amount of time our bodies store fat and decrease the time available to burn it. Because of this inverse relationship with insulin, increased carbs in your diet not only make you fat, but they also make you stay fat, even if you are eating less calorically than you need.

Carbohydrates are broken down into glucose, and glucose triggers insulin. Monitoring your carb consumption is more important than a trendy diet. It is a tool to stay ahead of your health. Your insulin factory will not be in overdrive and cells will stay sensitive to the hormone messengers that let your body know when you need energy. Furthermore, you will avoid both short- and long-term negative health implications.

How Well Our Cells Listen: Insulin Sensitivity

How quickly glucose is cleared from your blood is important. When your system is optimal and your cells are listening to the hormone messenger, insulin, excess glucose is removed quickly.

This means insulin is doing its job. Insulin is taking the fuel available and sending it into cells (muscles, liver, or fat) for immediate use or storage. Consistently high glucose levels, however, tire out your pancreas (your insulin factory) from all the extra work and dull the cells' ability to listen to the message insulin sends. As a result of this communication breakdown, insulin doesn't perform its job as quickly or effectively.

The result: glucose is not dealt with properly. Instead of being transported into the cells to be used for energy, the glucose remains in the blood stream making mischief everywhere from our skin to our DNA.

When glucose has a chance to hang out in our blood, instead of being filed away, it can stick to proteins in the body and form advanced glycation end products (AGEs). AGEs do exactly what the acronym implies, they age you. Too much excess glucose circulating makes you look older faster. And the glycation of collagen is implicated in the formation of wrinkled skin.

But that's not all. The effects of excess circulating glucose are more than skin deep. When excess glucose is processed, a by-product is created called a reactive oxygen species (ROS). In order to remain harmless, this ROS must be neutralized by antioxidants. However, we eat so much sugar and so little nutrient-dense foods that our bodies no longer have the antioxidants to neutralize these little devils. Overwhelming the body's defense system, these ROSs are free to damage cells, including our DNA. Long-term exposure to oxidative stress is involved with many diseases, including accelerated aging, Alzheimer's, Parkinson's, and chronic fatigue syndrome. It's especially hard on cells with slow turnover, such as joints and eyes, and can affect mobility and vision.

We want a diet that keeps our pancreas out of overdrive, and our cells listening to insulin. We don't want too much insulin—the fat maker—around.

If we are smart about our carbohydrate consumption, we can avoid many of the negative effects of high glucose levels. Choose slow-burning fuels such as greens, broccoli, cauliflower, and the sweet potato. They give you the energy you need without the bad effects of a rush of glucose through your system.

Normal cell

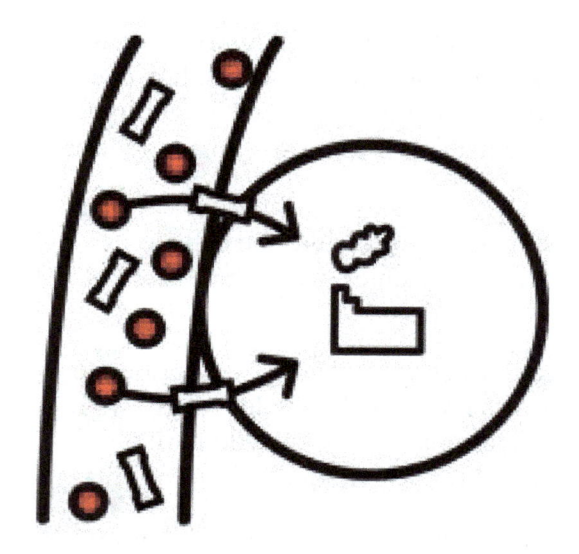

- Insulin is doing its job, allowing glucose to flow into cells when excess is in the system.
- Glucose fuel is utilized effectively by the cell, which goes about its business with energy steadily coming in and depending on cell type, going out.

⬤ GLUCOSE   ▯ INSULIN

Insulin Resistant Cell

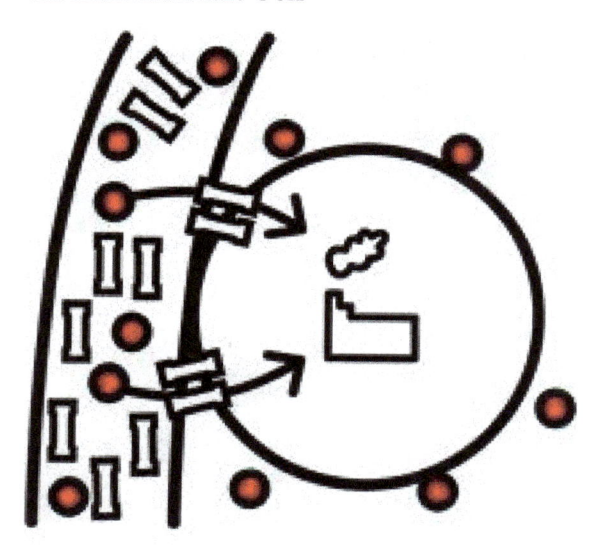

- Cells require additional insulin to store glucose, sending the pancreas into overdrive.
- Some glucose cannot make it into the cells and globs around the cells, causing oxidation problems.

Beyond Insulin: An Introduction to Cortisol

While controlling insulin is paramount for long-term health and easily within our power, insulin is not the only chemical messenger that affects our waistline. Stress causes more than just annoyance, it triggers the hormones adrenaline and cortisol, which affect how you store and release fat.

Cortisol is an important "get-moving" hormone, allowing us to get up and about after a long nightly fast. It prepares our bodies to deal with whatever is in the environment as soon as we open our sleepy eyes. When cortisol circulates, it tells cells to release glucose. This glucose is used to fuel muscles and to get us going, jump-starting our body until we can provide it with more energy in the form of food. Thus, our body produces cortisol in a natural cycle. Throughout the night, we ramp up cortisol production. When we wake up, it is naturally at its highest. During the day cortisol levels decline until they reach their lowest point in the early evening.

In addition to cortisol, adrenaline is another hormone that signals the body to release glucose. Adrenaline is called to action to help meet physical demands in a dangerous world. Adrenaline evolved to alert the body to flee or fight whenever the environment was hostile. Adrenaline was a brilliant adaptation. It arms each cell with loads of fuel, in the form of glucose, to respond to any threat, whether by running away fast or fighting hard. This glucose surge makes our brains think and react intelligently and gives our muscles the energy to perform well. Under these conditions, even fats and proteins are quickly metabolized into energy. When faced with a threat, the circumstance—feast or famine—doesn't matter. Adrenaline triggers the release of energy (glucose) into our blood to be victorious.

TOO MANY EXTENDED CARDIO WORKOUTS AND METABOLIC BEAT-DOWNS MAKE OUR BODIES THINK WE ARE RUNNING AWAY FROM LIONS.

In addition to triggering cells to pour glucose into our blood, cortisol and adrenaline also tell our body when to store or release fat. In the hunter-gatherer world our body was designed for, stress meant fighting or running away from predators. In terms of immediate survival, running away from predators ranked higher on the to-do list than eating, and a human on the run couldn't stop for a snack. So, thinking it is doing you a favor, stress triggers your body to hold on to fat as just-in-case storage.

Adrenaline served us well in a world where a saber tooth tiger could attack or woolly mammoths stampede. However, the functional role of acute stress (adrenaline) in the caveman world has morphed into unhealthy, chronic stress (cortisol) today. As soon as we walk out the door, we are faced with situations that put the body on alert. A car cuts you off. Crises arise at the office. Our days can be made up of ceaseless stressors. The body perceives each of these encounters as a threat. Accordingly, it keeps cortisol levels high and fat burning low.

Cortisol

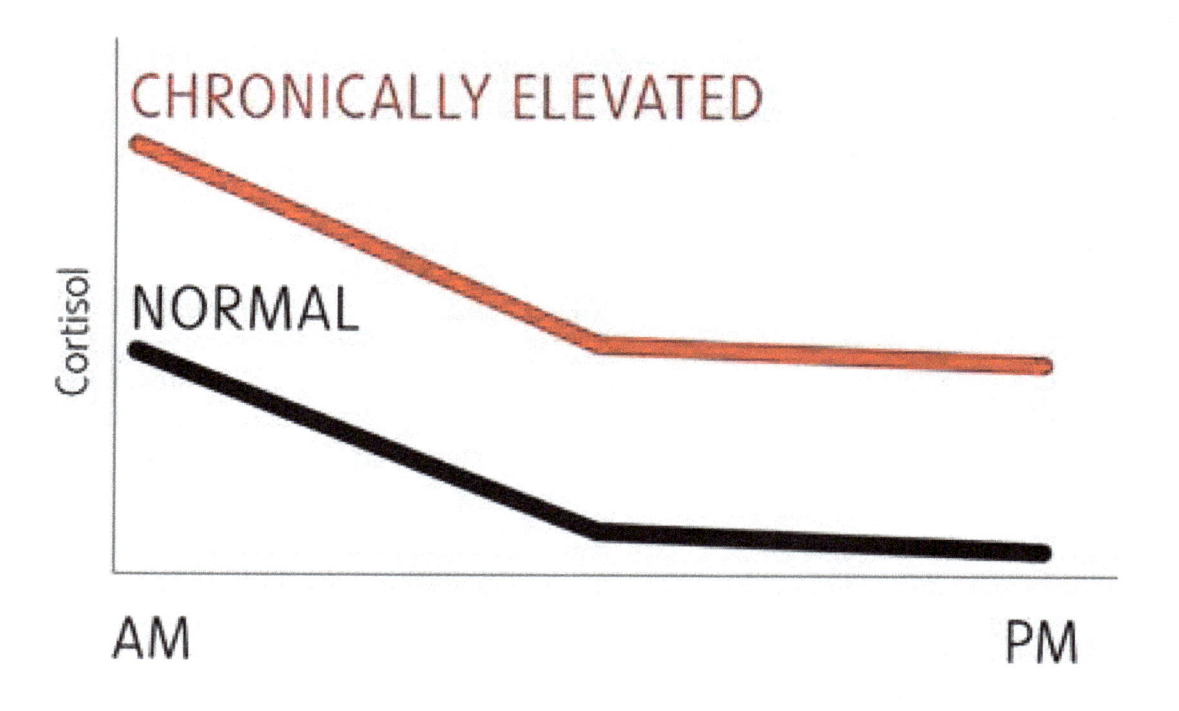

Cortisol (y-axis) vs **AM** to **PM** (x-axis)
- CHRONICALLY ELEVATED
- NORMAL

Too Much Exercise Adds to Stress (and Fat Storage)

Challenging the body in the right way can be healthy. Increased demands on the body call for a momentary bump in cortisol, which dissipates within an hour. When we choose the right type of exercise, this momentary bump can fuel activity that stimulates our muscles and bones to become stronger. It can also result in an overall reduction of stress post activity.

However, our body reads too much challenge as a stressor. To our body, excess exercise is the equivalent of running away from lions. Running away from lions is stressful (read: more cortisol). While our body was designed to deal with bouts of stress, we were not designed to deal with chronically high levels. While you think you are doing yourself a favor by "burning off calories" with your one-hour treadmill sessions every day, your body thinks it is doing you a bigger favor by holding tight to the emergency fat fund. The work you are putting in may be counteracted by the cortisol circulating in your system as a result of your overzealousness.

Beyond your waistline, high levels of stress from daily life, compounded with constant intense exercise, can be a recipe for disaster. If over the course of years you consistently overtrain—always pushing for maximum effort or until failure—you can put your cortisol factories in overdrive. Gone unchecked, our adrenal glands become overworked and can no longer keep up with demand. This is called adrenal fatigue.

When our hormone factories are tired and worn out, our body is not helped by the challenges in life. We no longer see gains in performance, and we feel tired, sluggish, and unmotivated. More time at the gym won't help you get over this fatigued state. The only thing that can help you recover is rest.

When It Comes to Food: Think Satisfied, Not Full

Imagine a pot. When empty, it has room for something to be put in it. When full, it has no more capacity. When applied to our bodies, "empty" means we are hungry, and "full" is supposed to mean we are not hungry. Volume is what fills up the pot, so we assume that volume is also what fills our stomachs and signals us to stop eating. But, it has happened to the best of us: we can still feel hungry even after we have finished a large meal. If your belly is full, why are you still hungry?

The term "full" has the wrong denotation; it should be replaced with "satisfied." Satisfied describes a state where a person feels satiated and no longer compelled to eat. The desire to eat more is gone.

Satisfaction does not have to do with the volume of food occupying the stomach. A person can feel satisfied and not be "full." Conversely, a person can be full without being satisfied. If satisfied is the state that we want to achieve, how do we get there?

SATIATED DESCRIBES A STATE WHERE A PERSON FEELS SATISFIED AND NO LONGER COMPELLED TO EAT. WHEN YOU CONSUME PROTEIN AND FAT, THE DESIRE TO EAT GOES AWAY. WHEN YOU CONSUME CARBS THE STOMACH CAN BE FULL BUT NOT SATISFIED, TELLING YOU TO EAT MORE.

TIPS FOR MAKING THE HORMONE CORTISOL WORK FOR YOU:

AVOID FOODS THAT SPIKE BLOOD SUGAR Fast rises in glucose are followed by subsequent crashes. When blood sugar dips below baseline, your body gets worried that it is starving. In response the body revs into gear with a stress response to get glucose to cells fast. Instead, eat fats and proteins, which fill you up by producing the right hormonal cues without the stress of the roller coaster ride.

AVOID CONSISTENT CARDIO WORKOUTS TOO MANY EXTENDED CARDIO WORKOUTS and metabolic beat-downs make our bodies think we are running away from lions. Running away from lions makes our bodies stressed, and when this stress is chronic, it causes our bodies to conserve potential energy by storing fat. How much exercise is too much? That depends on you and what your body can tolerate. Check out the guide to self-experimentation to find out what is right for you.

SLEEP IN A DARK ROOM Sleep in a blacked-out room. Too much ambient light while sleeping does not allow the proper reset of hormones at night.

AVOID BRIGHT LIGHTS BEFORE BED Avoid computer screens, TV, and other bright lights. Bright lights late at night make our bodies think summer. Summer means winter is coming. Winter means less food. Less food means we need to store more fat.

BEWARE OF SUPER-LOW CARBS IF YOU ARE AN ATHLETE In order to increase the breakdown of proteins and fats into fuel, the process (gluconeogenesis) up-regulates cortisol. This means extra stress on the body. Athletes who train hard benefit from having some source of quality carbohydrates, such as sweet potatoes, in their diet.

MEDITATE TO DE-STRESS YOUR LIFE Modern life is busy and full of demands. Take time to slow down, breathe deeply, and be present. Small efforts to reduce stress levels in the body can go a long way.

The Signal of Satisfaction: Introduction to "Enough-to-Eat" Hormones

Fullness of the stomach does not signal that our body is satisfied. This is why we can be stuffed and still feel compelled to eat. Instead, it is hormones, the body's communication tools, which signal us to eat or stop eating.

Hormones are made in a variety of locations throughout our body. One hormone we have talked about, insulin, is made in the pancreas. Other hormones are produced in the thyroid, hypothalamus, or reproductive organs. The biggest hormone factory is our digestive system. From beginning to end, our gut is one large endocrine system. It is a complex sensory tool that passes on information about what is going on throughout the body.

The foods we put in affect the messages that circulate in the blood. Our gut communicates to our body the answers to questions like: "Is it time to eat or stop eating?" "Is food abundant in the environment or is it scarce?" "Is it time to store up for winter?"

Hormones produced in our gut and throughout our body regulate our appetite according to the relationship between energy intake and metabolism. They tell our body when to "eat more" (the hormone ghrelin) and "when to stop eating" (hormones such as leptin, peptide YY, cholecystokinin, glucagon-like peptide 1, and oxyntomodulin).

When it comes to regulating our energy, most of us have a good sense of when we need to eat. When to stop is the more challenging problem. The key to putting the fork down is in the "stop eating" hormones, especially leptin. In today's normal everyday diet, those messages are lost in translation. However, when we eat what we are designed to eat, the message of when to stop comes through loud and clear.

THE KEY TO PUTTING THE FORK DOWN IS IN THE "STOP EATING" HORMONES.

When we eat the right foods, the "stop eating" hormone messengers are produced in the gut. Foods such as protein and fat stimulate the hormone production and help us feel satiated. When we eat these foods, our body gets busy processing the nutrients for immediate needs and short-term storage. Other foods, such as grains and sugars, do not produce the same response in the "enough-to-eat" hormones, leading us to serve ourselves unneeded seconds.

What we eat is not the only factor that affects "enough-to-eat" hormones. When we are stressed, our bodies hedge by preparing for the worst-case scenario. This means having enough stored energy to face a potential threat. Thus, we are stimulated by stress to eat more and store more. This stress can be a result of the demands of modern life. It can also be caused by something as simple as one night of bad sleep. When we don't get enough sleep, our appetites are seriously affected, triggering our bodies to reduce the production of leptin and increase ghrelin. This is why, when we are tired, we eat more and don't stop when full.

Leptin Resistance and the Dangers of Never Feeling Full

In addition to being produced in the gut, "enough-to-eat" hormones are also secreted by adipose (fat) tissue. When we eat large amounts of the wrong foods (bad carbs, sugar, grains, etc.), excess sugars are sent to fat cells for long-term storage. As we stuff ourselves with unhealthy food, the rush for space becomes so great that the storage units (fat cells) find themselves in danger of not keeping up with demand. They produce elevated leptin to tell the body to stop sending nutrients their way. The more fat we have, the louder the leptin message. Under normal conditions, this would make us feel satisfied and stop eating, but excess leptin can have a neutered effect.

Moderate amounts of "enough-to-eat" hormones help us feel comfortably satisfied. However, in the case of leptin, more of a good thing is not better. A modern diet with highly-processed carbs (sugar, fructose, and grains), chronic stress, and lack of adequate sleep combine to result in high levels of leptin. Just as our cells stop listening when too much insulin is present, our body stops listening when there is too much leptin.

WE ARE STIMULATED BY STRESS TO EAT MORE AND STORE MORE.

With chronic exposure, our bodies no longer hear the "I'm full" message. Over time, leptin cannot pass the blood-brain barrier that allows us to translate a hormonal message into action. As a result, the "I'm full" message doesn't make it to the control center—we find ourselves eating and eating and never feeling satisfied. Even worse, thinking that we need more food, our brain compels us to eat more. It's a vicious cycle, making weight loss difficult.

Hearing the "Enough-to-Eat" Messenger Loud and Clear

The foods we eat affect the hormones controlling our appetites. We need to make sure we are eating the foods that cause the right amount of "enough-to-eat" hormones to make us stop eating rather than the foods that produce so much our brains tune the message out.

Here are a couple of tips to make "enough-to-eat" hormones work for you, not against you:

- Eat proteins and fats that stimulate "enough to eat" hormones.
- Avoid foods that cause spikes in sugar and subsequent overproduction of leptin.
- Get adequate sleep.
- Work to lose the fat that overproduces leptin, causing dangerously high levels that lead to resistance.
- Avoid "grazing." Eating constantly can elevate leptin levels abnormally.

MORE THAN A LUXURY: THE IMPORTANCE OF SLEEP

The Guinness Book of World Records tracks all sorts of crazy, world-defying achievements, including longest free fall, sword-swallowing, and glass-eating. However, one world record will no longer be found in this tome of human achievement—sleep deprivation. Why did they stop recording this fact? Because lack of sleep is darn right dangerous.

More than a luxury, sleep is an essential biological function. Without it we don't function optimally. The problem? Most of us don't get enough sleep. Here are a couple of compelling reasons to get more shuteye.

SLEEP HELPS REGULATE YOUR APPETITE Two main hormones control our appetite, ghrelin and leptin. Ghrelin tells us to eat. Leptin tells us to stop eating. When we don't get adequate sleep, our hormones become imbalanced. Our level of leptin (the "stop" hormone) decreases by 18 percent. At the same time, our level of ghrelin (the "go" hormone) increases by 28 percent. When we are sleep deprived, we have a greater appetite and eat more. Not only are we hungrier, but we also crave high-carbohydrate foods.

SLEEP AFFECTS YOUR DECISION MAKING One bad night of sleep changes our brain's ability to function. Our prefrontal cortex, which controls logical reasoning, shuts down. The result—we are no longer capable of making good decisions. Choices like going to a gym or eating healthy foods become more difficult. This fatigue is apt to lead us down the wrong path.

SLEEP CHANGES THE WAY YOUR BODY PROCESSES SUGAR If we eat right and don't get enough sleep, all our hard work is for naught. Lack of sleep affects the way our body processes sugar and changes our body's glucose metabolism. With a glucose metabolism that is suffering, insulin production increases and our body stores fat more easily. Just a few days of sleep deprivation can lead the body to enter a prediabetic state.

SLEEP AFFECTS PERFORMANCE Children who sleep more score higher on IQ tests. For the rest of us, sleep affects our ability to complete simple and complex tasks either mental or physical. One night without sleep leaves us performing as if we were legally drunk at a blood alcohol content of 0.08.

SLEEP AFFECTS STRESS Cortisol is the hormone in our body that signals stress. While it has some important day-to-day functions, this messenger can get carried away with its charge, that is, to protect us in times of danger. Adequate sleep is required to control this hormone so it is working for us not against us. When we don't sleep enough, we produce more of this hormone. To ensure the body's survival, cortisol signals our cells to store fat and, instead, we burn muscle. All that wasted gym time! In addition, high levels of this stress hormone make us ravenous, so we eat more.

WHAT YOU CAN DO ABOUT HORMONES FOR OPTIMAL HEALTH:

KEEP YOUR PANCREAS OUT OF OVERDRIVE by minimizing exposure to foods that cause quick rises in blood sugar.

EAT FOODS THAT INCREASE INSULIN SENSITIVITY, such as the sweet potato and cinnamon.

PREVENT YOUR BODY FROM GOING INTO STRESS MODE by eating on a regular schedule and not skipping meals in times of stress.

INTERMITTENT FASTING CAN BE BENEFICIAL, but never do it in periods of stress in your life.

CHAPTER TAKEAWAY

Too often, people think that only diabetics need to w(orry?)
"healthy" people who eat diets moderate in sugar ca(n?)
become resistant to the hormone and forcing the p(ancreas?)
additional insulin in the bloodstream is visible to
converted to squishy fat as our cells become le(ss?)
send.

The other hormone to understand is cortisol, the s(tress?)
or at the gym, inspires adrenaline to flood into your bloo(d?)
stress, you body wants to hold on to its potential energy fat. v(?)
high levels of this hormone, weight loss becomes difficult.

What you eat and how you live your life affect the hormones circulating in y(ou?)
Controlling your carbohydrate intake is the best way to regulate blood sugar and (?)
levels in check. If we eat too many simple carbs, too much insulin is released, which le(ads?)
Moderate amounts of sweet potatoes give us the satisfaction of eating carbs without the nega(tive)
effects of a spike in insulin. This nutritious treat also makes cells more sensitive to insulin
without taxing your pancreas, the insulin factory, with extra work.

CHAPTER 5

INFLAMMATION: WHEN FOOD BECOMES FOE

THE WAR WITHIN: HOW FOOD FOSTERS REBELLION IN THE GUT, AND HOW WHAT WE EAT CAN BE THE BIGGEST ALLY OF HEALTH

The Double-Edged Sword of Inflammation: An Introduction

Inflammation is an important part of the healing process. When you sprain an ankle, it gets swollen. This reaction is the work of your body's healing agents mobilizing and rushing to fix the problem. Most people only think of this visible, "acute" reaction when they think of inflammation—the redness, the swelling, the tenderness. In contrast, the inflammation that we can't see, present in the blood, has the most influence on our health and waistline.

Acute inflammation is a good thing that helps heal our bodies. But, if the body is always in healing mode, it experiences chronic or constant inflammation, which is damaging. When our systems experience nonstop inflammation, our bodies are constantly fighting invaders. The relentless siege taxes fortifications. While the body is fighting on one front, resources are not available to fight new threats like disease and infection. We get sick more often. One of the most common sources of chronic inflammation is our food. With the wrong foods, chronic

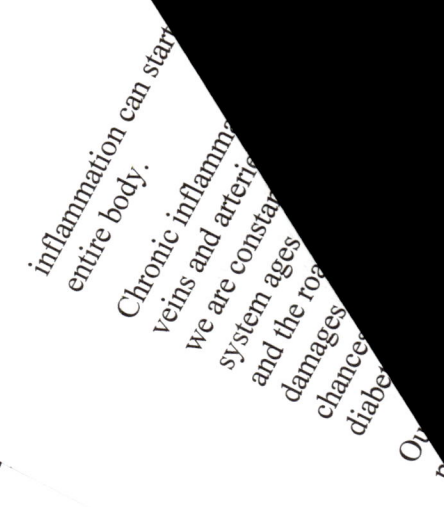

...in our digestive system and move into the bloodstream and through the...

...tion can be likened to emergency fire trucks that go out to fight problems. Our ...s are the roads that take these emergency vehicles around our body. But when ...tly bombarding our system with heavy equipment and nonstop travel, the transport ...and wears out. These transport highways—veins and arteries—become less elastic ...d system gets smaller. Chronic, high inflammation makes you age faster. It also ...your DNA, making it more prone to replication errors. These errors increase the ...s that cells may become cancerous. Also, chronic inflammation increases the risk of ...es, high blood sugar, and weight gain.

...r brain needs glucose to do its job. Inflammation in the intestine lowers efficiency and ...revents glucose from getting to hungry cells. The result? Your body feels a nutritional deficit and tells you to eat more. To quickly feel better, we are compelled to eat bad foods that get processed quickly. These bad foods cause more inflammation, perpetuating the vicious cycle.

Some causes of acute inflammation are out of our control, such as our bodies fighting bacteria or viruses, or healing from injury. However, chronic inflammation can be controlled. We should avoid foods that cause inflammation and load up on foods that help fight it.

Food as a Friend or Foe

The body needs to keep the bad stuff out to be safe from invaders that harm and destroy. At the same time, supplies from the outside world are needed to keep going. To get these nutrients, it is necessary to allow some exposure to destructive elements. To deal with this problem, the body separates incoming material into food friends and food foes. Food friends are needed reinforcements that fuel and replenish the body. Food foes cause damage and harm.

Food friends and food foes are separated in the small intestine for their different journeys. The small intestine acts as a checkpoint and barrier on the road, letting the good nutrients through to the bloodstream and hungry cells, and keeping the bad stuff moving along its way to elimination from the body.

Anti-Inflammatory	Moderate Inflammatory Foods	Egregious Inflammatory Foods
Broccoli	Potatoes	Wheat
Brussels sprouts	Legumes (beans, peas, lentils)	Rye
Cabbage	Corn	Barley
Kale	Rice	Oats
Sweet potatoes	Watermelon	Sugar (white, brown, fructose)
Grapefruit	Bananas	Alcohol
Berries	Honey	Artificial food additives
Herbs	Quinoa	
Almonds	Canola oil	Deep Fat Frying
Walnuts	Vegetable oil	Peanuts
Olive Oil		Trans fats
Fish oil		
Coconut oil		
Meat (grass or pasture raised)	Beef and Poultry (grain fed)	Soy
Fish (wild or line caught)	Dairy	Tofu
Omega-3 eggs		Processed Meats (salami, bologna)

When our small intestine is overrun with bad food, the body mobilizes to keep the bad stuff out. Inflammation comes to the rescue, fortifying the small intestine to prevent the absorption of toxins into the bloodstream. But, less absorption area for the bad also means there is less absorption for the good nutrients our bodies need. Inflamed surface cells in the intestine cut down the surface area from about 2 million square centimeters to 2,000 square centimeters. The body's overzealous attempt to protect against food foes also can cause injury. Innocent, helpful cells are caught in the crossfire, preventing them from transporting good foods.

Unable to get the needed supplies through the inflamed intestines, our body tells us that we ate the wrong food through stomachaches, gas, diarrhea, cramps, and bloating. We feel groggy and have less energy. We often don't understand the message and, as a result, we do not heed the warning.

Inflammation from food foes does not stop in the small intestine. Despite the body's best efforts to keep the bad stuff moving toward elimination, food foes sometimes slip through the checkpoint and enter the bloodstream. Once again, the body sends inflammation emergency vehicles through the bloodstream to deal with the threat.

Under Siege: Sneaky Foods and Their Effects

What is the difference between food friend and food foe? Food friends give you an advantage. Food foes weaken your defenses.

Like us, plants have evolved to reproduce and spread their seed. Different plants have different strategies to do this. Some plants, like fruit, have developed a "give a little, get a little strategy." Fruits give critters a scrumptious, energy-rich flesh. In exchange for this delicious treat, plants expect some seeds to be carried to new places and deposited in fertile packets to propagate and grow. It's a mutually beneficial arrangement.

Wild grasses—predecessors of wheat, rye, oats, barley, millet, and rice—developed a different strategy. Their seeds needed to reach maturity before spreading to the wind. To deter small rodents from chowing down before seeds had a chance to mature, grains included self-defense mechanisms. These self-defense mechanisms caused irritation in digestion, making small critters sick and deterring them from demolishing the plant's ability to reproduce. The grass's defenses worked, at least for small animals. When larger animals started to belly up to the grain buffet, however, those self-defense mechanisms no longer had the same level of success in driving them away.

During human digestion, grains are broken down into a variety of proteins, including some called lectins. While the body is trying hard to keep food foes out, lectins disguise harmful molecules. The disguise, a type of molecular mimicry, makes the body think food foes are our friends. Our body lets these molecules into the bloodstream, where they can bind to almost any tissue and wreak havoc. Different grains and legumes contain different lectins: soybeans contain SBA, peanuts PNA, and kidney beans PHA. One of the nastier forms of lectin is wheat germ agglutinin (WGA) found most commonly in the wheat kernel. These are large protein/carbohydrate hybrids that do not get broken down in digestion. When soaked or cooked the effects of these lectins are minimized. However, wheat gluten, or specifically, gliadin (a type of protein that makes up gluten) does not break down in cooking. Gliadin is a prime food foe suspect.

THE BODY TRIES HARD TO KEEP FOOD FOES OUT. DISGUISED AS FOOD FRIENDS, LECTINS BREACH THE BODY'S DEFENSES AND ENTER THE BLOOD STREAM WHERE THEY WREAK HAVOC.

Once the enemy combatants are circulating, our body figures out the guise and sends an inflammation emergency response team to fight. But there's a problem. This enemy protein looks similar to the body's good proteins. When the emergency crews are fighting, they can mistake good guys for bad guys and hose them down in the confusion. For many people, this results in high levels of inflammation. Extreme cases result in autoimmune disease, such as rheumatoid arthritis or multiple sclerosis.

The effects of these large protein hybrids don't stop there. As large, unauthorized proteins glom on to the gut lining, they break down the defenses and cause intestinal permeability. Partially digested food spills into the bloodstream. This is called leaky gut. The more breaches in our gut, the less capable we are of extracting the sugars, proteins, and fats we need from our food friends.

OUR BODIES DON'T HAVE MEGAPHONES. THEY SPEAK SUBTLY.

Getting Our Gut Back On Track: Learning to Listen to the Message

Our bodies don't have megaphones. They speak subtly. The body tries to communicate its messages through bellyaches, diarrhea, stomach cramps, and fatigue. But since most people consume inflammatory food foes daily (wheat, oats, barley, rice, corn), these messages are ignored. Other times the list of symptoms is so extensive, diagnosis can't be definitively determined. Patients instead are given an unspecific verdict of "irritable bowl." While silently suffering internally, we see around us more cases of obesity, arthritis, heart disease, and autoimmune diseases. One culprit is raging, unseen inflammation. Cleaning up our diet through consistent good eating repairs the damage and gets the system in working order again. People who embrace a paleo diet (a diet that cuts out these offenders) are rewarded by feeling good. Try a paleo diet for a month and see if you look, feel, and perform better.

For those who want to cheat, cheat the smart way. Know how foods fight back and which ones pack the most harmful punch. Wheat gluten is one of the most harmful. In addition to being bad for you on a daily basis, a cheat meal containing gluten can cause damage that your body takes all week to recover from depending on your gut and immune function. So when the time comes to cheat, choose other grains for cheat meals and avoid gluten all together.

WHAT YOU CAN DO ABOUT INFLAMMATION FOR OPTIMAL HEALTH:

ELIMINATE FOODS FROM YOUR DAILY DIET THAT FIGHT BACK, including grains, legumes, and, most importantly, wheat and its processed component gluten. Make sure to check labels; just like sugar, gluten is sneaky and makes its way into many packaged foods, including some brands of sweet potato fries!

WHEN YOU CHEAT, CHEAT THE SMART WAY. Avoid wheat all together and instead cheat with less aggressive grains, such as corn and rice.

BE AN EDUCATED HEALTHCARE CONSUMER. Stay informed. The science of chronic inflammation is not given its due.

CONSIDER MAKING GOOD FOOD CHOICES FIRST TO ADDRESS HEALTH PROBLEMS. Don't jump straight to treating symptoms; treat underlying problem first.

CHAPTER TAKEAWAY

Chronic inflammation is the body's reaction to bad foods. It taxes our systems and makes us feel ill. Chronic inflammation is also the foundation of serious diseases later in life, such as rheumatoid arthritis, osteoporosis, and Alzheimer's disease.

How is it prevented? Avoid the foods that cause chronic inflammation, especially wheat and other grains. Unfortunately, these foods are the foundation of the Western diet, so they can be hard to eliminate. Sweet potatoes are great substitute and a food friend we can rely on.

Also, listen to the body. Often, the foods our gut reacts to are so commonplace that we think uncomfortable bloating or cramps are normal after every meal. Use your diet to surround yourself with food friends instead of food foes. Eating foods that don't fight back keeps our small intestines in tip-top shape to absorb only the good nutrients and reject the bad.

CHAPTER 6

ACTIVITY: MORE IS NOT ALWAYS BETTER

MOVING AND FUELING FOR MAXIMIZED BENEFIT

Move, Move, Move

Optimal health demands that we do what our bodies are designed to do. This means eating what we are supposed to eat and moving. Our primal forefathers had to earn what they ate. Natural periods of activity (searching for food and running away from predators) and rest were built into daily life. In today's affluent societies, physical activity must be sought out. If we want to be healthy, we have to make the choice to move.

Exercise does wonders for our bodies. Our hearts are strengthened when we make them work hard. Stronger hearts are more efficient, even when resting. When we challenge our muscles, they also get stronger and more toned. Our bones become denser and more resilient when we lift weights, preventing osteoporosis down the road. Some experts say exercise even boosts cognition and makes us
smarter.

With stronger muscles, denser bones, a healthier heart, and better-functioning brain, our health and performance is optimized. Additionally, exercise changes the way nutrients are partitioned on a cellular level. When we exercise, our cells get better at dealing with insulin. Exercise is an important tool in combating glucose issues, and, in some cases, exercise can even help reverse the effects of type 2 diabetes. Whether we are standing instead of sitting at our work desks, taking short walks, or lifting weights, activity is an important part of our genetic makeup.

Being active is a way of life, not something you check off the to-do list every day. Adding activity need not be a daunting task. With little forethought, increasing movement can be a pleasurable addition to life, as well as a tool for making you healthier. Here are a couple of ways to get in the swing of things.

STRATEGIES FOR INCREASING ACTIVITY:

SET REALISTIC GOALS Adding activity can be as simple as increasing how much you move or walk every day. If exercise has not been a part of your routine, start small. Choosing goals that are attainable will give you early success and help you avoid the painful side effects of exercising too hard. Build up your strength and tolerance gradually.

WALK MORE Cars are convenient. It is easy to forget that we can easily walk to accomplish some of our errands. Put your car in park and try doing some of your errands on foot or bike. Enjoy the journey, not just the destination. Walking will do as much for your happiness as it does for your health.

MAKE ACTIVITY FUN When we enjoy what we do, we are likely to do it more often. Choose activities that are enjoyable. Whatever it is, whether jumping on a trampoline, hiking in the woods, or playing kick ball, fun exercise can help make activity seem like a break and less like a chore.

SEEK COMMUNITY Working with others can provide extra encouragement, accountability, and motivation to push further. Find others who share the same goals and set regular times to get together for your activity of choice.

DON'T COMPARE YOURSELF TO YOUR GLORY DAYS It is easy to compare yourself to years ago, when you played sports in school or were in tip-top shape. Don't hold yourself to the same standards you held when you where eighteen. Your body changes and so should your expectations.

Choosing the Right Activity for Your Biology

The health benefits of activity are undeniable. Just as our bodies function best with certain foods, they also function best when we include activity. But we need to make sure the exercise we are choosing provides the right type of stressors. Some stressors stimulate the body to become stronger while other stressors weaken the body. For most people a moderate level of activity is enough to achieve optimal health without overtaxing the body.

Extreme athletes, who constantly push themselves to their limits, need to be careful about providing the proper rest for their body. For hunter-gatherers, work and rest came in cycles. Seasons forced our early ancestors to slow down. Hunting large game allowed them to rest between meals so they were not working hard every day. While demanding, life was not always strenuous from morning to night.

Today we live in an athletics-obsessed culture. Extreme sports, endurance training, and one-upmanship in physical feats are the norm. To hear a coworker recount his marathon or triathlon in the office on a Monday morning is not uncommon. This culture is a recent phenomenon. Ask your parents what they did with their spare time when they were younger. They probably weren't working out at the gym.

In the 1960s heavy physical activity was thought to be bad for you. But as an article in the New York Times reported, by the 1970s this view had lost popularity in favor of the "new conventional wisdom—that strenuous exercise is good for you." This was followed in the 1980s with the rise in popularity of running and the introduction of new types of aerobics. Cities and towns all over the country built sporting exercise stations on public trails, broadcasting the message that working out is important to health.

We should not let exercise trendiness get in the way of what is healthy for our bodies. Extreme fitness (ultra-marathons, Ironman triathlons, etc.) is fun, but we need to make sure our exercise provides good stressors that make us stronger, rather than weaker, by avoiding adrenal fatigue and excess inflammation in the body. Sometimes this means backing off for a time and choosing activities that are less stressful.

The Dangers of Exercise: Getting Fat while Getting Fit

The Ironman Triathlon is a 2.4-mile swim, followed by a 112-mile bike ride, and capped off with a 26.2-mile run. Completing an Ironman with no training is not possible. Ironman athletes train hard, two to four hours a day, burning a huge amount of calories. Even with all their extra training, we see many chunky people at the starting line, even some who are fat. These demanding sports do, of course, produce plenty of svelte bodies and opportunities for some to show off their six packs. But even in these elite athletic circles, the body on the cover of Men's Fitness is the exception rather than the rule. So, what gives?

Most of these endurance sports are fueled by carbs, and lots of them. Check out a pit stop at any marathon. You will see sports gels, Gatorade, bananas, and other carb-tastic goodies that would send any four-year-old into a covetous tantrum. These "foods" are effective at delivering sugar into cells, which is why they fuel our elite athletes. But, their kick comes at a cost. Even during a period of strenuous training, increased carbs still have the same results for super-athletes as they do for the rest of us. Carbs affect insulin levels, encourage fat storage, spark inflammation, and impair immune function.

If even elite athletes who work out prodigiously are fat, those of us who are ordinary gym-goers should take note. No amount of exercise is going to give you carte blanche to eat whatever you want. Fueling smartly is imperative, especially when appetite is increased from exercise. You don't want to get (and/or stay) fat while you are getting fit.

Someone who is lean and doesn't exhibit metabolic degradation can eat sweet potatoes post-workout. For someone who has to lose fifty pounds, it would be best to keep the carbs low until they can regain some of that insulin sensitivity.

For Athletes: Smart Timing of Carbs to Augment Performance

Most casual gym goers will do just fine with smart fueling and carb monitoring. Intense activity for athletes demands nuanced fueling for performance and recovery. Physical activity demands more energy from cells. We can use our hungry cells to our advantage. Eating quality carbohydrates can be a great tool for attaining our athletic goals, whether we want to fill the tank without getting a spike of insulin, demand more performance from our bodies, or fuel smartly during extended physical activity.

Carbs Post-Workout: Not for Everybody

Store shelves have a growing range of products for post-workout promising improvements in body composition and gains in performance. However, casual gym goers and athletes need to be wary of these claims. Filled with carbs, these products (sports drinks, recovery shakes) are not for everyone.

Those who are overweight should stay away from flooding their body with extra carbs. Excess fat is a sign that insulin is not doing its job. If this is you, give your cells a break to get your body on track. Consume only 20–40 grams of protein post-workout. Once you have leaned out, you can then add in carbs.

USE CARBS TO ACHIEVE BETTER PERFORMANCE

Priming the pump with a bit of pregame fuel can be the difference between a personal record and a workout that's only so-so. The extra glycogen (glucose) coursing through your arteries just might give you that little extra bit of performance that you have been chasing. Lighter foods in small quantities will do the trick, like a portion of baked sweet potatoes.

Again, know your body. Some people feel nauseous if there is food in their stomach when working out. For others, small amounts of carbs are just the thing to get going.

SMART FUELING DURING EXTENDED WORKOUTS

We need fuel or our bodies stop. Our bodies naturally have enough energy stored in the muscles and liver to sustain activity. Once we've exhaust our stored energy, continuing exercise hurts unless we refill the tank. For extended activity, a steady refuel supply is essential to keep going and going and going.

To refuel on-the-go most athletes will reach for a shiny silver pouch of liquid fuel. Don't be fooled. These little space-age wonders are full of funky ingredients. If you plan ahead, you can make your own sports gels that are in line with your diet values. Check out the recipes at the end of the book for some examples of homemade sports gels.

A side note: some people's palates change, and they prefer less sugar during extended periods of exercise. Play around with a variety of flavors for exercise fuel. When you turn your back on packaged "performance" foods, you might find that you can better give your body what it needs—especially if that is more salt and less sweet.

DON'T BE FOOLED BY SHINY, SILVER POUCHES OF LIQUID FUEL. THEIR KICK COMES AT A COST.

POST-WORKOUT FUELING: HOW TO GET CARBS WITHOUT SPIKING INSULIN

Incorporating carbs the right way can help get needed energy to muscles without the negative effects of insulin. One of the best times to incorporate carbs into your diet is post-workout. When we move hard, our bodies use the energy stored in liver and muscle cells. When we are done, our cells are left starving and screaming for nutrients. We want to take advantage of our cells' hunger window and deliver them the protein and carb s they crave to refill depleted stores. If we do this soon enough after exercise, we don't get a hit from insulin. Score!

Some say the optimal time for this carb- and protein-rich refuel is less than fifteen minutes after a workout. It's still a good time at thirty minutes out, but the clock is ticking. After an hour, your body will be back to its baseline for responding to elevated glucose in your blood.

Plan ahead if you want to take advantage of this window of opportunity. Your post-workout fuel needs to be handy right when you finish your last rep. This snack should include carbs to feed cells and protein to repair them. Stretching, debriefing a workout with your friends, or driving home does not count as workout time. Be smart. Have what you need on hand to refuel so you don't have to rush or skip other important post-workout measures, such as mobility training and stretching.

TAKE ADVANTAGE OF THE CELLS HUNGER WINDOW AFTER WORKOUTS SO YOU CAN SHUTTLE GLUCOSE INTO CELLS WITHOUT A HIT OF INSULIN.

How Does the Sweet Potato Fit In?

If we are defining optimal health as healthy food + balanced hormones + low inflammation + right activity, the sweet potato is the smart food to support us.

As a healthy food, nutritious sweet potatoes provide complex carbohydrates that can fuel your cells. Sweet potatoes can take the place of bad carbs such as grains and legumes.

As for balanced hormones, sweet potatoes are a quality smart carb. Reasonable amounts of sweet potatoes do not cause spikes in insulin, and they can even help encourage insulin sensitivity in the cells. Furthermore, unlike other foods, sweet potatoes allow the hunger messenger hormones to tell us when to eat more or when to stop.

To keep internal inflammation low, a smart carb like the sweet potato is a valuable tool. It helps repair your gut and, unlike wheat or corn, it doesn't cause your system to react and fight against it. With sweet potatoes you can have access to all of the energy and nutrients without any of the damaging side effects of bad carbs.

Finally, sweet potatoes can be used to support the right kinds of activity for optimal health. Using sweet potatoes smartly, athletes can take performance to the next level by timing consumption before, during, or after workouts to help reach fitness goals.

Sweet potatoes can be a valuable tool in your arsenal for optimal health. Incorporated into your diet, you can use the sweet potato to fight many of the health problems that are widespread today. In a world of detrimental carbs, nature has given us the smartest carb of all—the sweet potato.

QUICK TIPS FOR ATHLETES ABOUT THEIR CARB INTAKE:

Balancing carbs and endurance fitness is a tricky tightrope. Here are a couple of rules that will keep you on the right track:

BE PICKY ABOUT YOUR CARB SOURCES
Wonder products may leave you feeling like you just strapped on rocket boosters to fly to the moon, but nature makes fuel best. Stick to complex carbs from real foods so you don't burn up shortly after liftoff.

STAY AWAY FROM FRUCTOSE
Due to its high sweetness level, a lot of sports products use this sugar to keep calories low. But, you want your sugars to go straight to your muscles, not your liver.

KNOW WHAT YOU NEED
When you are adding extra carbohydrates to fuel extended activity, know your tolerance. The goal is to refill the tanks without going overboard and triggering insulin responses and fat storage mechanisms. Track yourself. Monitor how you feel. Use trial and error to tweak your plan for optimized performance.

BE HONEST ABOUT YOUR GOALS
Reasons abound to engage in endurance-type sports or training. For some, it's just fun. For others, it's a way to manage stress at home or at work by making their body simulate that running-away-from-lions feeling. For many people, weight loss is the goal. If you are in this last group, be smart and diligent. No amount of working out is going to give you a free pass to eat what you want. Even with intense training, diet needs to be the foundation of a healthy lifestyle. If you aren't getting good nutrition, no amount of running is going to shed those extra pounds.

MAKE YOUR OWN OCTANE
Make your own gels and recovery formulas. Sports supplements are expensive in terms of cost and health. Formulating your own fuels, tailored to your activity, is easy and will result in a better-quality product. Again, know yourself. If you are metabolically compromised (overweight or experience insulin insensitivity) simple carbs in any form can spike insulin, especially in the fast-delivery liquid or gel formats.

ACTIVITY YOU CAN DO FOR OPTIMAL HEALTH:

INFUSE YOUR LIFESTYLE WITH EASY MOVEMENT, like walking, hiking, or throwing a Frisbee around. Make it a shared goal with your friends.

FOR MORE INTENSIVE ACTIVITY, CHOOSE EXERCISE THAT IS RIGHT FOR YOUR BODY, reducing stress instead of causing it. Listen to your body. Take a rest if your routine is doing more harm than good.

FUEL SMART. Don't fuel hungry muscle cells with empty carbs or fructose bombs. Choose proteins and complex carbs that won't spike your insulin.

EXPERIMENT WITH TIMING OF YOUR ACTIVITY FUEL to increase performance and health. Do your carb and protein refuel within thirty minutes of your workout.

DON'T BE SWAYED BY MARKETING PRODUCTS AIMED AT ATHLETES, which are full of sugar. Instead consider nature's power food—the sweet potato—as your smart source of energy.

CHAPTER TAKEAWAY

Our bodies are designed to go through periods of activity and rest. While our ancestors had to be active in order to catch food and avoid predators, today's modern conveniences allow a passive lifestyle that robs us of many of the essentials of optimal health. To restore our bodies to health, we must intentionally infuse our lives with movement—anything from simply walking or standing to playing sports or going to the gym with friends.

But be careful! Some people overcompensate and forget that periods of rest are also natural and essential. The right activities strengthen our muscles, bones, brain, and circulatory system, but too much can lead to excess stress and inflammation. Just as our ancestors did, back off and give your body a break every once in a while.

With increased activity, our bodies demand more fuel. But don't think that you can just work off anything you put into your body. Even in athletes, too many carbs lead to the vicious cycle of insulin production, resistance, and fat. Make good food choices—before, during, and after you exercise—to support strong peak performance, optimal recovery, and a lean physique.

Part III

YOUR BODY, YOUR RULES

AN OPTIMAL HEALTH COOKBOOK

CHAPTER 7

A STEP-BY-STEP GUIDE TO OPTIMIZE YOUR HEALTH

—

TESTS, TOOLS, AND TRICKS TO HELP YOU LOSE WEIGHT, SEE HIDDEN INFLAMMATION, MANAGE STRESS, AND OPTIMIZE PERFORMANCE.

A note to the casual reader This chapter is written for people looking to monitor and develop a highly personalized lifestyle for optimal health. If the techniques described here seem too involved or invasive to you, don't sweat it—skip straight to the recipes for sweet potato power!

The Importance of Making Your Own Rules

Want to make changes in weight but trendy diets failed you? Want to be proactive in keeping your good health? Exercising but not seeing progress? Eating right but not seeing results? Want to head off or reverse disease and illness? While general guidelines set you on the road to the finish line, they sometimes fall short in taking you all the way.

Each of us has a unique biology. Our tolerances for foods, stress, and activity vary. We are in different stages of life. General guidelines don't factor in our specific make-up or environment. Our bodies are dynamic biological systems that are constantly changing. What you did three years ago is not what you should be doing now. We need to adapt to see continued results.

At the same time, the health world around us is complex. General guidelines don't always address a person's specific needs. The health care system can be sick-care not well-care. The sick often get the most attention with their immediate problems. Those who want to be proactive about their health may not receive the desired attention.

Armed with science and a few tools, you can become more knowledgeable about your own health. With a commitment to listen to your body, observe, and act on results, you can develop guidelines that work specifically for you. You can also track health markers in order to address and treat warning signs before they become problems. How can you do this? By building self-knowledge through monitoring and experimentation.

Self-monitoring and experimentation are valuable ways to gain a better understanding of your body and create the guidelines that work for you. While the effort may deter some, those who choose to engage enter into a fascinating realm of self-discovery. You will understand your body and learn to serve it better. This approach can help answer questions such as:

- How do I lose weight?
- How can I better listen to the messages my body sends?
- Why do I still carry fat if my diet is dialed?
- What foods most likely make me fat?
- What markers can I look for before I get sick?
- How are my cells responding to insulin today?
- What are the effects of eating too much fruit?
- How can I tell if I have hidden inflammation in my body?
- How do I know whether or not the exercise I am doing is causing more damage than good?

We Are All Experimenters

Whether we realize or not, we have all participated in self-experiments. When we eat a new food or try a new activity, we are experimenting. If we enjoy what we eat, we will eat it again. Conversely, when we have negative reactions or don't enjoy the food, we choose to pass the next time. In either case we do something and observe the outcome. We modify our behaviors now that we are better informed.

This chapter helps you approach your health in new ways by providing you with the tools for obtaining and tracking how far you have to go to reach optimal health. Experiments range from simple observations that require nothing more than counting to tests that require a doctor's order and lab expenses.

Don't be intimidated. You don't need every test. And you don't need to track for a long period of time. Monitoring is not to manage an illness (sick-care). We use monitoring to optimize wellness (well-care). Think of it as your own adventure for optimal health. Pick and choose what is most relevant or interesting and dive in. The results can be enlightening and life changing.

Setting Up Experiments

For those seeking frequent insights about their body, self-monitoring and experimentation can be revealing. It's not hard. A little planning and foresight is all that is necessary. Here are some simple tips:

- Set up experiments ahead of time. Be explicit about what you are trying to learn.
- Limit testing to one or two variables at a time. For example, perform the test at the same time of day, under the same stress levels, or with the same foods.
- Be curious. Look for anomalies in your data. Ask yourself what could be the causes? Develop and test your hypothesis.
- Before you draw conclusions, be critical of your data. Ask yourself if other factors could have had an influence on what you observed.
- Be clear about your assumptions. Does your data support or reject your underlying assumptions? If your data does not support your assumptions, how could your assumptions be wrong?
- Good science is repeatable. Try your experiment again.

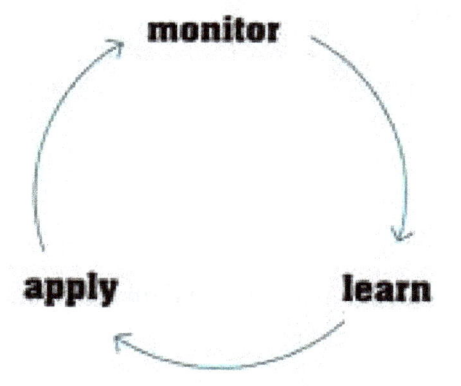

monitor → learn → apply → (monitor)

Self-monitoring does not have to be an ongoing process. In the context of well-care, monitoring is a tool to learn more about your body and collect insights that can be applied to improve life and health. What you monitor changes. The goal is to grow in your knowledge about yourself.

A Word on "Normal"

In this section, you will see the words "in range," meaning your numbers look good, and "out of range," meaning your numbers could use some improvement. The values and ranges you see will not always correspond with standard ranges. This raises the question: What does normal mean? Truth be told, normal is arbitrary, and it changes. Let's take blood pressure for example. Forty years ago medical schools taught that 100 plus your age meant normal. If you were 65, your blood pressure should be 165. Today your blood pressure has to be under 120 or you are in heart attack territory and need drugs fast! Cholesterol measures have changed too. As recently as 1962 the reference book for doctors Current Diagnosis and Treatment stated that normal cholesterol ranges between 150–280mg/L. Doctors today say values should be under 200mg/L.

While our standards have changed, clinical outcomes have not necessarily gotten better. Blood pressure and cholesterol metrics are the two most commonly cited indicators for heart attacks. More people monitor and treat them than ever before. However, 50 percent of heart attack patients have "normal" numbers of both cholesterol and blood pressure. Normal is not the sole predictor of future health.

To further confound the issue, most guidelines are based on the averages from a diverse population. As we know, the average population in a country like the United States is not the ideal specimen of health. Aspiring to be "of average health" would be like aiming for a C in your standard college course that grades on a curve. Instead, we should aspire to be in tip-top shape for optimal energy, performance, and long-term health. We don't just want to be told when we have a problem. We want to see red flags early and avoid problems altogether.

WE DON'T WANT TO BE TOLD WHEN WE HAVE A PROBLEM. WE WANT TO SEE RED FLAGS EARLY AND AVOID PROBLEMS ALTOGETHER.

As a result, the numbers given here as "normal" are based on optimum health and longevity. While some doctors will look at your numbers and say you are fine, you now have the tools to raise red flags for yourself. No one cares about your health more than you do.

QUICK GUIDE FOR EXPERIMENTS:

Here is a list of tests to run to help work on specific goals—from losing weight to optimizing performance.

TO LOSE WEIGHT

BEGINNER Count carbs and try to stay within a healthy range.
INTERMEDIATE Monitor baseline blood glucose levels with a glucometer.
ADVANCED Use frequent glucose testing to determine responses to meals, stress, and other variables.

TO TEST THE EFFECTIVENESS OF A NEW DIET

BEGINNER Track weight when changing a diet with tools such as the Withings Scale.

INTERMEDIATE Compare blood work before and after diet change (C-reactive protein to test inflammation levels, cholesterol panel, HbA1c).

TO DECREASE INFLAMMATION

BEGINNER Track carbs. Avoid inflammation-causing carbs (wheat, corn, and rice) by eating more anti-inflammatory sweet potatoes.

INTERMEDIATE Test inflammation levels with C-reactive protein test and avoid exercises that overly tax muscles.

ADVANCED Determine problematic foods that you don't tolerate through food elimination tests.

TO OPTIMIZE PERFORMANCE

BEGINNER Use basic indicators of look, feel, and performance to tinker with optimal carb levels.

INTERMEDIATE Monitor cortisol response from activities through "adrenal stress index testing" and plan more strategic exercise breaks before your body starts to wear out.

ADVANCED Determine optimal workout cycling and diet cycling based on specific performance goals.

Asking for a Blood Test and Working with Your Doctor

Some tests in this section require a doctor's order before the test can be done. Find a doctor who can help you gain the knowledge that you need and interpret the results. A supportive doctor can be a valuable ally. Ideas to keep in mind when working with your doctor:

ASK FOR WHAT YOU NEED. No one cares more about your health than you do. Speak up for what you want.

MAKE A LIST OF WHAT YOU WANT AND WHY. Have a clear, written list of the tests you want performed. You should have a succinct reason for each test in case the question comes up.

ASK AHEAD WHAT INSURANCE WILL COVER. Know your insurance company's reimbursement rules. Often more tests will be covered than you think. Many plans include routine blood work at least once a year.

BE PREPARED TO PAY CASH FOR TESTS. If insurance does not cover what you are asking or if you want results off the record, don't be afraid to pay out-of-pocket.

REQUEST PRICING AND SHOP AROUND. Before you get pricked, shop around for the best price. Costs range greatly between doctors' offices, standard pricing cost, cash price, insurance, walk-in lab facilities, and online. Before you decide, review the price list in the summary section as a good starting point.

EXPLORE ONLINE OPTIONS. Some tests don't require blood to be drawn. Test kits can be sent through the mail and save considerable cost. Also for tests requiring a blood draw, lab facilities with a trained phlebotomist can run tests. Look online at LabCorp or Quest Diagnostics. Call ahead to see if you need a doctor's prescription for a test.

DON'T BE INTIMIDATED THE FIRST TIME AROUND. Learning how to navigate the system for the first time is the hardest part. Once you set up a relationship with a doctor or a lab, subsequent visits will be easier.

FIND ANOTHER DOCTOR IF YOU DON'T GET THE SERVICE YOU WANT. Doctors are service providers. If they are too busy to provide the service you want, find someone who will.

"WELL-CARE" DOCTORS ENTER INTO A PATIENT'S CARE AS A PARTNER. THEY WORK WITH YOU TO OPTIMIZE YOUR HEALTH TO AVOID SICKNESS ALTOGETHER.

Choosing The Right Partner In Health

Conflicting opinions exist in the world. Doctors are no different. One doctor with the authoritative stethoscope draped around his neck may say lab values are fine, but his view may be from a perspective of diagnosing sickness, not optimizing wellness. "Sick-care" doctors look for results that diverge from the average and respond by prescribing a medication or making a blanket nutritional recommendation. "Well-care" doctors enter into a patients care as a partner. They will take basic lab results as a starting point and consider the whole picture. While a sickness-oriented doctor might look at high cholesterol results and say it's time to cut back fats, a wellness doctor looks deeper at the information, noting ratios of triglycerides to HDL and partial sizes in your LDL report. He may see that your cholesterol actually looks great.

Finding a well-care doctor is finding a partner in health. You are required to do your part. They curate knowledge, insight, and interpretation. Together the doctor-patient team works for the goal of long-term health. In many medical schools only a few hours of nutritional education are provided. To receive the most up-to-date information, you need to find a doctor who reads the nutritional literature, has the patience to critique efficacy studies, and sometimes the bravery to go against the grain of conventional wisdom.

Doctors also need to empathize with your underlying philosophies. This can be difficult. Some doctors are often more comfortable with standard approaches and an overreliance on medication remedies with pressures from insurance companies to go through high volumes of patients. Be stalwart in your search. Great practitioners are out there. Many doctors desire patients who are engaged and proactive with their health.

The right doctor or health practitioner will work patiently to optimize your health, utilizing medications as a last resort instead of a first line of defense. In addition, having the right partner will set you up for a long-term relationship that will serve you well as the health data monitoring industry matures around us. Today people like you can collect and store more personal data than ever before, allowing you to track information, such as heart rate, blood pressure, activity levels, sleep patterns, diet, hormonal levels, and glucose. In the next couple of years, we will see patches that collect even more personal health data with even greater ease, perhaps in the form of little Band-Aids we wear on our bodies. This information is invaluable, but it is raw and subject to interpretation. We need doctors to serve as guides helping us unravel the results to understand what it all means. Finding the right doctor now will set you up for success later, as the tools get better and more ubiquitous.

CHECKLIST FOR FINDING THE RIGHT WELL-CARE DOCTOR:

The time will come when you need to call in a professional to reach the bottom of an issue. Here is a list to keep in mind:

- Thinks holistically across systems of the body and across disciplines
- Explains issues thoroughly, problems, and points of interest
- Points you to resources that further your own knowledge
- Reads primary studies and talks to you about them
- Expects you to follow recommendations
- Supports patient self-monitoring and experimentation
- Uses medication as a last resort

For those seeking to find a sympathetic doctor or health guide, check out the Paleo Physicians Network. This network is a great starting point to find doctors who are deeply committed to prescribing good living and eating habits instead of pills.

Category: Food, Hormones (insulin)

Difficulty: Easy

What you need: Access to nutrition data, pencil and paper, or other tracking tool

Cost: Free

CARBOHYDRATES

RECALIBRATING OUR CARB-O-METER: COUNTING CARBS TO RESET NORMAL

WHY THIS TEST
Dietary carbohydrates directly influence insulin in your body. Limiting carbohydrates avoids food explosions in your system and evens out energy.

WHAT YOU CAN EXPECT TO LEARN

- Determine general range of carbohydrate consumption.
- Learn the carbohydrate load of your favorite frequent foods.
- Uncover hidden carbohydrates in diet.

BACKGROUND
Quick, how many calories in a banana? What about carbs? Even if you knew the calorie count, chances are you missed the carbs question. Given the obsession with calories, it is no surprise most people need assistance to come up with the amount of carbs in a given food.

The number of carbs in food doesn't rank at the top of the memory bank. Beyond the obvious carb culprits, secret carbs weasel their way into our diets through foods, such as ketchup, salad dressing, and mayo. Most of us don't even count those as carbs. When we do keep mental tallies, we forget to include the hidden carbs in unassuming foods and beverages like coffee drinks and alcohol. Chances are our counting mechanism needs some recalibration.

Eat lots of bad carbs and look fine? Don't think you are off the hook. Just because your body does not respond to poor food choices by gaining weight does not mean your body won't feel the hurt. The skinny girl who eats whatever she wants may be slim and trim, but she runs a high risk of other hidden consequences from bad dietary choices. If she wants to have a baby, for example, she may not get pregnant because chronically high insulin can lead to hormone imbalances that result in infertility.

WHAT TO DO

1. To reset your carb-o-meter, track your food for two weeks using a computer program or phone app.
2. Use any program that shows more than just calories and goes into the macronutrient breakdowns of fat, proteins, and carbs.
3. Tap and Track, for instance, allows you to save common meals and input data on a computer or phone while on-the-go.

Collecting data is only part of the process. Take time to learn from your observations. Each night look at your numbers. How did you do? Any carb culprit surprises? What was your daily carb intake?

INTERPRETING DATA

Here are some helpful guidelines to interpret your carb measurements:

Danger zone: >300
Weight gain zone: 150–300 grams (U.S. recommended daily allowance)
Optimal carb intake for effortless weight maintenance: 100–150 grams
Weight loss sweet spot: 50–100 grams
Ketosis: <50g

By the end of two weeks of tracking and observing, you will have an intuitive sense of how many carbs you are eating and what foods are the culprits.

The Primal Blueprint Carbohydrate Curve

- 300+ g: Danger Zone
- 150–300 g: Insidious Weight Gain
- 100–150 g: Effortless Weight Maintenance
- 50–100 g: Weight Loss Sweet Spot
- 0–50 g: Keto/I.F.

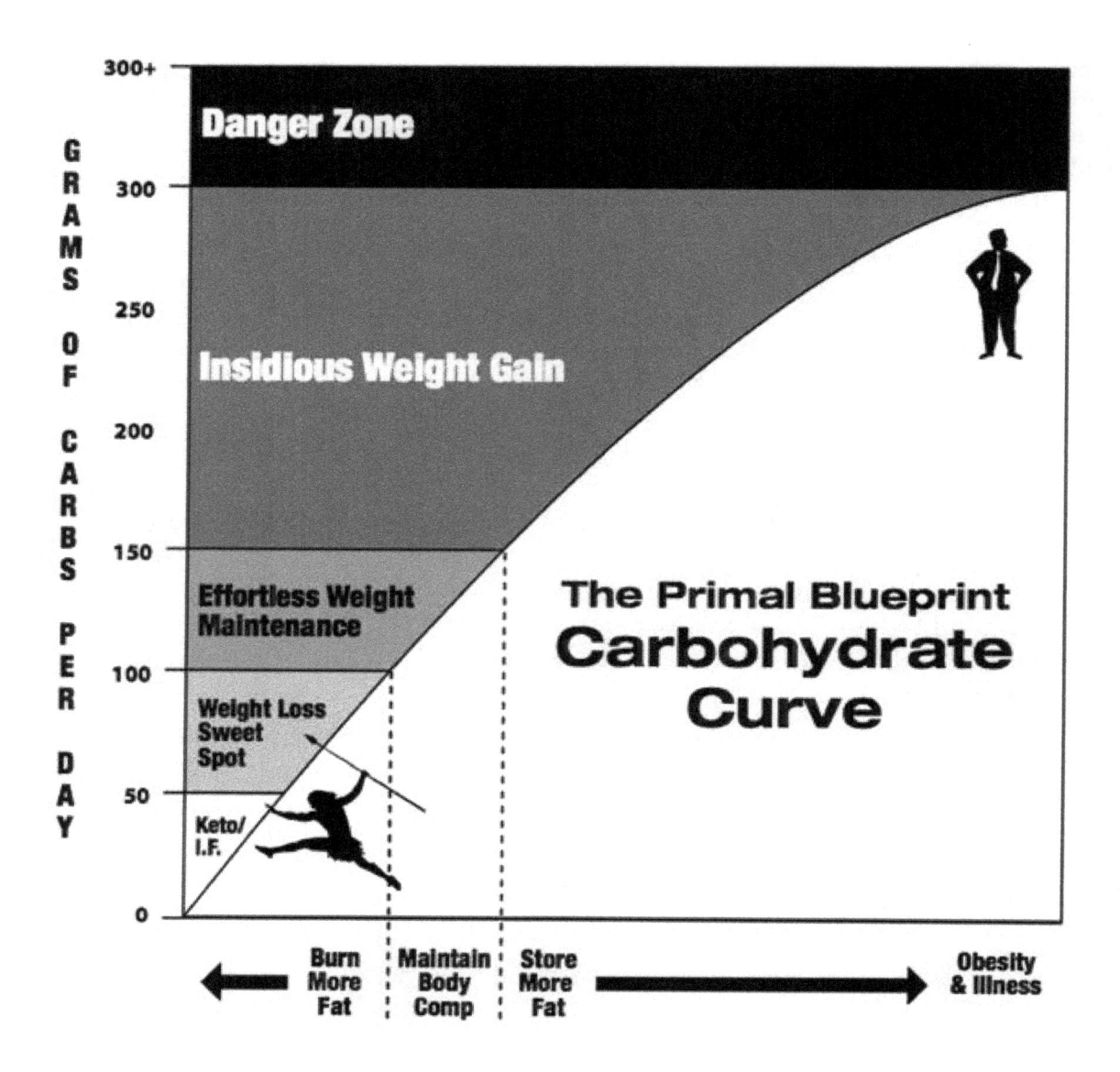

Horizontal axis: Burn More Fat ← Maintain Body Comp : Store More Fat → Obesity & Illness

After working with hundreds of clients one-on-one, Mark Sisson summarizes his findings with his Carbohydrate Curve. Check out more about Mark and his practical guides for living a low carb life on his blog, 'Mark's Daily Apple.'

Category: Food, Hormones Activity

Difficulty: Intermediate

What you need: Self-awareness, pencil and paper, access to nutrition data

Cost: Free

CARBOHYDRATES

OPTIMIZING CARBS: HOW YOU LOOK, FEEL, AND PERFORM TO REFINE CARB INTAKE

WHY THIS TEST

Our bodies want to run at optimal levels. This means feeling good, being alert and rested, and staying disease free. Anything outside of optimal is a "symptom" and is your body's way of trying to communicate. In order to be responsive and fix underlying causes, we have to tune into our body's frequency.

WHAT YOU CAN EXPECT TO LEARN

- Develop carb guidelines based on your own needs, not general ranges.
- Identify messages your body is trying to communicate through its physique, performance, and feelings.

BACKGROUND

Your body tells you when you are not eating properly or taking proper care. Begin by keeping a record of how you feel throughout the day. This will help you pay more attention to your body, hearing what it says more clearly. Common symptoms are: cravings; energy swings; headaches; soreness; hunger; not sleeping through the night; waking up tired after a full night of sleep; pain; acne; joint stiffness; unprovoked anxiety; poor attention; and, for women, irregular menstruation.

Listening to your body is the best tool you can give yourself for optimal health. Once you start hearing the message, you can tweak your diet to make the changes that your body is asking for.

The chart opposite is an example of how you might want to organize your observations so they can be helpful tools in formulating the magic numbers that work best for you and your biology.

WHAT TO DO

For a week keep a Food and Symptom Log. Record as much as you can even if you do not think it is food-related. To get started here are some questions to ask yourself.

- How many carbs am I eating a week?
- How do I feel during a workout, physically and emotionally?
- What am I craving?
- How does my skin look?
- How fast can I recover from a workout?
- When am I hungry?
- What is my attention span?

When you have done this for a week, sit down with your data and review the results. Based on the chart, what is your body trying to communicate? Are you eating too many or too few carbs?

OUR BODIES ARE NOT "SET IT AND FORGET IT" MACHINES. WE NEED TO TUNE INTO OUR BODY AS IT CHANGES. THE MORE YOU PAY ATTENTION, THE BETTER ABLE YOU'LL BE TO INTERPRET THE MESSAGES IT SENDS.

INTERPRETING THE DATA

Deciphering the data is case specific. On the following pages are a couple of examples to illustrate a variety of situations and how the chart can be utilized to interpret symptoms of too many or too few carbs.

Symptoms of Too Many Carbs

Look	Feel	Perform
Overweight	Lethargic / Afternoon energy slumps	Poor recovery and soreness post workouts
Acne*	Depressed / Mood swings / Mental Fog	Sore Joints
Bloated	Limited attention span	
	Anxiety / Hyper	
	Lack of focus	
	Sugar cravings / Midnight hunger pains / Food obsession	Poor sleep patterns / Fatigue even after getting a full night of sleep

Symptoms of Too Few Carbs

Look	Feel	Perform
Lean or fat	Sluggish	No motivation to train
	Depressed / Flat personality	Muscle fatigue / Slow reaction time, i.e. no snap in muscles
		Slow recovery

Indicators of Right Amount of Carbs

Look	Feel	Perform
Lean	High energy	Muscle energy
Clear skin	Consistent energy levels / Attentiveness and focus	Motivation to move and work out
	Mental sharpness	

*While not all acne is a sign of too many carbs, most acne can be reduced with a paleo diet, which is dairy and sugar free. This acne elimination methodology works for most cases.

SYMPTOMS LOG

- Does not feel hungry in the morning
- Feels hungry shortly after eating
- Has trouble concentrating in the afternoon and feels in a daze

- Extra weight around the midsection
- Carb count 350 grams/day in sample diet

Case Study #1—Andrew

Andrew works in an office and spends most of his day sitting at a desk. Four to five times a week, he goes to the gym and runs on a treadmill after work. He runs less often when busy with his job. He considers himself a health-conscious eater.

When Andrew wakes up, he is not hungry. So he does not eat before heading out the door. On the way to the office, he picks up a cup of coffee with cream and sugar. Mid-morning he eats something quick, such as instant oatmeal or a banana that he keeps in his desk. His favorite work time is the mornings when his brain is sharp. By 12:30 PM he is ravenous. Lunch is a sandwich with chips and iced tea or a hamburger with fries. By mid-afternoon he is hungry again. He feels tired and groggy. He loses focus. He is less productive and easily distracted. To power through he drinks a bottled frappuccino or eats food stocked in the office kitchen—cookies, yogurt, or candy. After work he heads to the gym. Returning home, he stops for a burrito with extra veggies and black beans for dinner. Later in the evening, he might forage in the fridge for something tasty. He often eats a bowl of cereal before turning in.

He is six foot one and 210 pounds. Even though he works out, he has a soft, round tummy. Since he regularly works out and thinks he eats healthy, the extra weight does not bother him. Andrew considers the extra pounds his natural set point.

Looking at the day, we can identify some of the symptoms Andrew is experiencing. Correlating these symptoms and numbers, we can use the graph to determine how Andrew is doing. Andrew is eating too many carbs.

CARB RX: Andrew should eliminate many of the high-carb culprits from his diet by focusing on natural food from nature (meats, vegetables, nuts, seeds, some starch, little fruit, no sugar) instead of processed foods. Breakfast needs to be a priority to get his day started right. He should not drink sugar beverages. With his light running on the treadmill, Andrew should seek to eat fewer than 100 grams of carbs a day until he leans out and symptoms improve.

SYMPTOMS LOG

- Working out is a chore
- Muscles are sluggish
- Does not see progress in workouts
- Hypersensitive about gaining weight
- Carb count 45 grams/day in sample diet

Case Study #2—Chris

Chris weighs and measures all of his food and lives a strict, low-carb, paleo diet. He has a cheat meal once a week, usually on Saturday night. He is committed to CrossFit four to five times a week. He has been doing this for two years, come rain or shine. In the last couple of months, he has not seen improvement in his performance, despite putting in the time. These days dragging himself to CrossFit seems to take all the self-discipline he can muster. He feels tired and sluggish. His muscles no longer feel like they are full of energy. Chris is convinced his cheat meals are to blame so he cuts them out.

Chris wakes up early to make his breakfast. He has four eggs with half an avocado, sometimes adding hot salsa for flavor. Chris packs his own lunch and loves to eat chopped salads with 5–6 ounces of chicken breast. For a snack he will have 27 almonds and 2–3 ounces of grass-fed beef jerky. Dinner is often a quick chicken stir-fry with onions and peppers. Jerky and nuts are his snack food. When he feels particularly famished, he will eat almond butter straight from the jar.

Weight conscious, Chris is lean with a solid build and 9 percent body fat. He used to be 25 pounds heavier and worked hard to shed the extra pounds. Fearing he will gain it back if he takes a break, he stays hyper-vigilant on his workouts and diet. Chris feels he would rather under-carb than over-carb.

Using the chart, Chris looks at his symptoms and carb numbers each day to determine how his body is responding. He needs to be flexible and listen to his body, increasing his good carbs into a more comfortable range.

CARB RX: Although Chris's carb numbers are in the optimal range, based on the way he is feeling, he is not getting enough carbs. Even though Chris is currently lean, his history of being overweight implies that his body does not tolerate carbs well. He needs to incorporate carbs after a workout, when the body can take advantage of non-insulin mediated glucose uptake. Eating a smart carb like a sweet potato after a workout will help him achieve increased performance while not gaining weight.

Case Study #3—Sarah

Sarah is thirty-two years old and a dedicated athlete who trains twice a day for a triathlon. She wakes up early in the morning and grabs an energy bar as she is running out the door to bike before work. Sometimes in her long rides, she "hits the wall" (runs out of energy). Fearing she is not consuming enough calories, she feeds herself on her bike ride with a packet of carb gel every thirty minutes.

Despite working out two to three hours a day, Sarah is still a bit thick in her stomach. Most people would not say she's fat; but she considers herself "skinny fat." She wishes she could cut back the calories but figures that since she is working out so much she needs the energy. The alternative is running out of steam more often. Sarah consistently gets adult acne. While she considers herself too old for acne, she attributes it to sweat from her intense workouts.

When done with her morning workout, Sarah will eat a banana and eggs before heading to work. At work she feels energized in the morning. Since Sarah makes her own lunch, she is not tempted to go out. One day she goes out with some colleagues at lunch and has a Cobb Salad. On that day her office celebrates a birthday. She indulges in a slice of cake, thinking she's earned it and will be burning off the calories later. After work she heads to the pool for a swim, fueling up with a Gatorade. Finished, she heads home for a dinner of salmon with green beans.

SYMPTOMS LOG:

- Runs out of energy frequently
- Cravings

- Depression
- Acne
- Carb count 185 grams/day in sample diet

She refrains from dessert after dinner; but she can't stop thinking about sweets. She obsesses over cupcakes and ice cream. Most of the time she doesn't give in; once or twice a week she does. Sarah has lots of energy but frequently feels a little down. She can't point her finger at anything that would make her feel this way. Work is going well and socially she has more friends than ever from her new training. But, something still feels off.

Using her daily carb number, Sarah determines her carbs are high. Based on her activity level, though, she thinks her carb consumption is appropriate. She looks at her symptoms to determine if this is the case.

CARB RX: Sarah should clean up her carbs by eating more natural foods to fuel her activities. Processed sugars from performance products, if not tolerated well, can lead to many of the problems she is experiencing, such as acne. Adult acne is a symptom of inflammation in the body. Cleaning up the quality of carbs can also help with depression. Eating nature's foods, as we are built to do, can be one of the first lines of defense against the blues.

IF YOU WATCH THE SCALE, A TWENTY-POUND GAIN DOES NOT SNEAK UP ON YOU. IF YOU WATCH YOUR GLUCOMETER, METOBOLIC DERANGEMENT WILL NOT SNEAK UP ON YOU EITHER.

The New Scale: Introducing the Glucometer

The glucometer is like a weight scale but better. We are all familiar with weight scales. Even if we don't use them every day, we have a general idea about our weight. We understand how the scale works. We put on weight; the scale goes up. We lose weight; the numbers go down. Pretty simple.

In addition to measuring your weight with a scale, other important metrics and tools are helpful. A twenty-pound gain does not sneak up on you if you keep tabs on your weight. If you keep an eye on blood glucose levels, other problems that go unnoticed and result in chronic disease won't sneak up on you either.

Your blood glucose level is important. Since glucose triggers insulin, blood glucose levels are an indicator of how well your body is responding to this hormone. Are the cells still listening? Or are they tired of hearing the insulin message and starting to tune out? When you familiarize yourselves with the numbers, glucose can also tell you how your body is responding to the food you eat, such as whether the sugar/carb load of your diet is too high. If your diet is clear of blood sugar-spiking foods and your numbers are still high, this can be an indication of high levels of stress. Testing insulin requires a doctor's order, a skilled professional to draw blood, and some fancy equipment. In contrast, testing glucose is easy and can be done at home.

Today, blood glucose is tested with a glucometer, which measures glucose levels in a small drop of blood. A glucometer can be purchased over the counter at a pharmacy, usually for less than $15. It comes with a meter for reading results, lancets (small needles), and test strips.

GET TO KNOW THE HIDDEN RHYTHMS OF YOUR BODY AND THE LANGUAGE IT USES TO COMMUNICATE.

Those who feel hesitant about drawing blood, no matter how small an amount, fear not. Noninvasive glucose meters are on the way. Companies like Echo Therapeutics are developing needleless glucose monitors that read glucose levels through our skin with a Band-Aid-like patch. While these systems are out of the price range for most casual experimenters, we can look forward to lower prices and more tools using this ouch-free technology in the future.

As with the use of a weight scale, how often you use the glucometer depends on your goals. Testing a couple of nights in a row before bed will give a basic understanding of how your body is processing your daily sugar intake from the day. For those trying to gain a deeper understanding, lose weight, or tinker with their diets, checking five times a day for two weeks can provide useful information.

As with any new skill, time and effort are required before you feel confident testing and reading your glucose level. Be patient. A single prick can only provide a snapshot of data connected to a given moment in your life. It won't reveal a wealth of secrets. Over time, however, you will get to know the hidden rhythms of your body and the language it uses to communicate. Your glucose level is an easy place to go to translate a piece of that message.

HOW TO TEST BLOOD GLUCOSE USING A GLUCOMETER:

1. Purchase a glucometer starter kit at any pharmacy.
2. Kits come with a lancet (a small needle) to prick skin, test strips to read blood, and a meter to display results. Instructions may vary depending on the device. Familiarize yourself with the manual before proceeding.
3. Insert a test strip into the meter. When the machine is ready, it signals you to place blood on the test strip.
4. Using the lancet provided in the kit, pick an area on the tip of your finger that is free from calluses. With the tool provided, the needle will be injected shallowly into the finger to produce a small drop of blood the size of a pencil tip.
5. Dab the drop of blood onto the tip of the test strip device for analysis.
6. After 10–15 seconds your glucose level will be displayed on the screen.
7. Record your results.
8. Never share lancet needles.

HELPFUL TIPS

- Use different fingers to avoid callus buildup.
- If you don't get enough blood, try squeezing the tip of your finger before you prick yourself again.
- Sharp needles hurt less. To minimize the ouch-factor, change needles frequently.

- While you may be proud to be testing your blood glucose to optimize your health, be discreet about where and when you test. Many people dislike the sight of someone drawing blood in public.

Category: Food, Hormones

Difficulty: Easy

What you need: Glucose monitor and test strips, recording method

Cost: $

INSULIN

MY BODY'S RESPONSE TO ITS DIET: GLUCOSE TESTING END OF DAY CHECK-IN

WHY THIS TEST
Since glucose triggers insulin, with a simple test you can see how well your body is responding to this hormone. Taking tests a few nights in a row before bed provides a basic understanding of how your body is processing your daily carbohydrates.

WHAT YOU CAN EXPECT TO LEARN

- Discover how your body is dealing with glucose at the end of the day.
- Track trends inside your body over time.
- Spot warning signs before problems arise.

BACKGROUND
One of the simplest ways to check blood glucose is before bed. This glucose reading gives you a solid understanding of how well your body is managing your dietary carbohydrates throughout the day. Some practitioners tell you that glucose reading is best when the stomach is empty. However, before bedtime gives you more information on how your body is processing foods.

WHAT TO DO
1. Perform a glucose test nightly before bed for one week.
2. Record results.
3. The week of tests should be repeated every four months.

INTERPRETING THE RESULTS
If you weigh yourself only once, the number is meaningless. After weighing regularly, however, the measure becomes more meaningful. Just like weight, you want your blood glucose numbers to be in context and meaningful over time.

Some practitioners consider these ranges as a helpful guide for optimal health.

....

PRE-BED GLUCOSE (MG/DL)

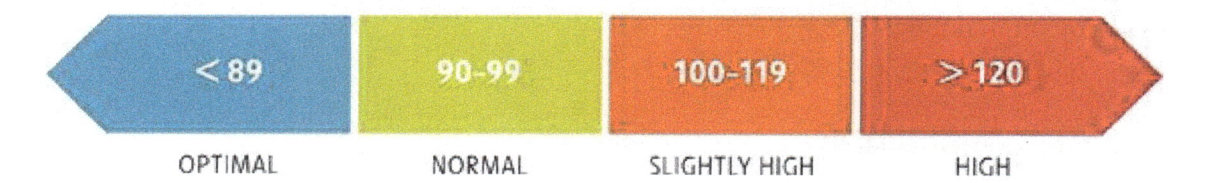

< 89	90-99	100-119	> 120
OPTIMAL	NORMAL	SLIGHTLY HIGH	HIGH

Consistently high glucose levels generally means high insulin levels. Even if you feel great right now, chronic exposure to high glucose is not good for long-term health. If your glucose is high and you aren't paying attention to your diet, don't be surprised. Our bodies were not designed to live in this contemporary Candyland of perpetual sugar and carbs. It isn't too late to take action, however; our cells are resilient. If we make changes early enough to our diets, our bodies can bounce back. Keep reading. You will find some good tools to manage your diet and create a plan that works for you.

WHAT FOODS WILL MAKE ME FAT: GLUCOSE TESTING RESPONSE TO FOODS

Your body is unique, so are the foods it can tolerate. While some might do well with sweet potatoes, fruit, or sweets, others might not. It is up to you to determine what foods give you healthy blood sugars. No matter what health messages are broadcast, if a food spikes your blood sugar over target ranges you should not eat it.

Using your glucometer you can develop what foods work best with

1. Take a baseline test
2. Eat only food you are testing
3. Take blood test 1 hour after eating

....

GLUCOSE (MG/DL) ONE HOUR AFTER MEAL

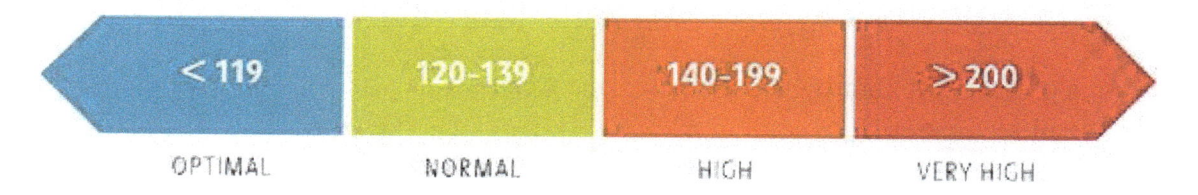

< 119	120-139	140-199	> 200
OPTIMAL	NORMAL	HIGH	VERY HIGH

your body.

HOW TO TEST

If blood sugar surges out of health ranges, don't despair. Try adding some fat to slow down digestion. Retake the test again a couple of days later. If values are still high eliminate foods from your diet all together.

Category: Food, Hormones

Difficulty: Intermediate

What you need: Glucose monitor and test strips, recording method

Cost: $

INSULIN

GET OFF THE SUGAR ROLLER COASTER: GLUCOSE TESTING THROUGHOUT THE DAY

WHY THIS TEST
The glucometer gives us new eyes to peer inside our bodies and check out what's happening. Learning to incorporate this simple tool into routines can develop our understanding of how we process the food we eat and how well our cells respond.

WHAT YOU CAN EXPECT TO LEARN

- Effects of different foods on your glucose levels.
- Manage energy throughout the day more effectively.
- Understand if you are actually hungry.
- Identify which meals lead to high glucose and insulin spikes.
- Familiarize yourself with personal glucose patterns.
- Reinforce good eating choices with data.

BACKGROUND
For those who are ready to dive into the data, this is a more involved way of testing glucose. Using a glucometer in the same way already described, test your blood five times per day. This is good for people learning to manage their glucose levels, optimizing carbohydrates during meals, choose the right foods for their bodies, and experimenting with their body's tolerance for sugars. We want glucose levels to be consistent throughout the day, providing a constant stream of energy to our body, while at the same time avoiding rollercoaster–like ups and downs.

WITH DATA, WE CAN BEGIN TO PIECE TOGETHER THE STORY OUR BODY TELLS.

WHAT TO DO

1. Perform an initial "fasting" blood test immediately after waking and before eating anything.

2. Do a second and third test two hours after breakfast and lunch, respectively.
3. Take a fourth reading immediately before dinner. Finally, take one more reading before bed.
4. Record all results and all food eaten.

Keep this testing regimen over a period of at least two weeks. Over this time period, you will become accustomed to your patterns.

INTERPRETING RESULTS

Reading the results is easy. Consider your fasting blood glucose to be the baseline. Two hours after meals, blood sugar will be higher but should be within approximately 20 points. Before dinner and before bed (this is assuming you are going to bed several hours after eating), blood sugar should be close to your fasting range from first thing in the morning.

If you have elevated glucose levels after meals, before dinner, and at bedtime, start adjusting your diet to see how you can get your numbers in order. Your goal is to have as consistent a reading as possible. When the glucose line doesn't move more than 20 points from fasting at any given test time, this means that you have a constant stream of energy throughout the day. You will avoid the mental fogginess, post-lunch slumps, and urges to take naps that plague almost all those who eat a normal, Standard American Diet.

Sit down with your data and do some analysis. Are your numbers sky high across the board? Think about what in your diet could be to blame. Is your diet low carb but the glucose numbers still seem high? If so, see the section about cortisol and stress. If you are stumped, find a doctor or other practitioner who will work with you to help you understand what's going on and why.

....

FASTING GLUCOSE (MG/DL)

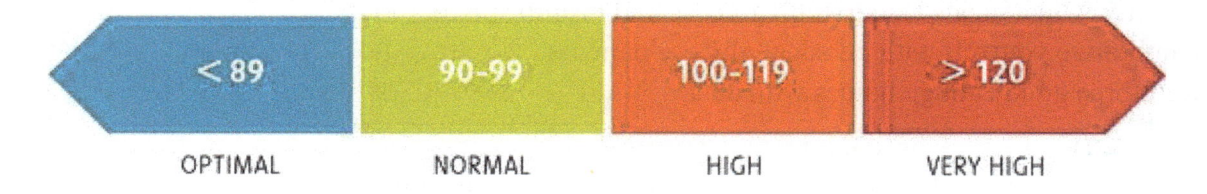

< 89	90-99	100-119	> 120
OPTIMAL	NORMAL	HIGH	VERY HIGH

....

GLUCOSE (MG/DL) ONE HOUR AFTER MEAL

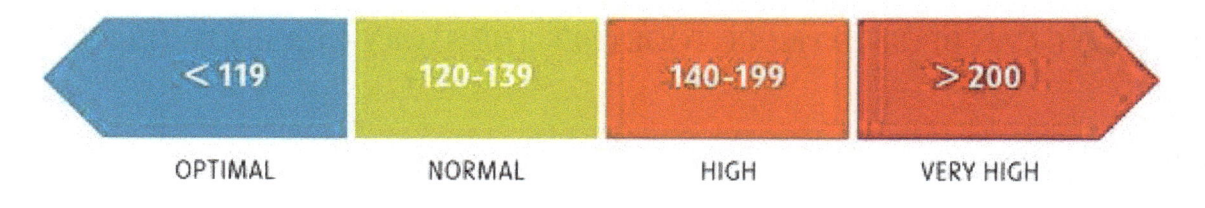

< 119	120-139	140-199	> 200
OPTIMAL	NORMAL	HIGH	VERY HIGH

....

GLUCOSE (MG/DL) TWO HOURS AFTER MEAL

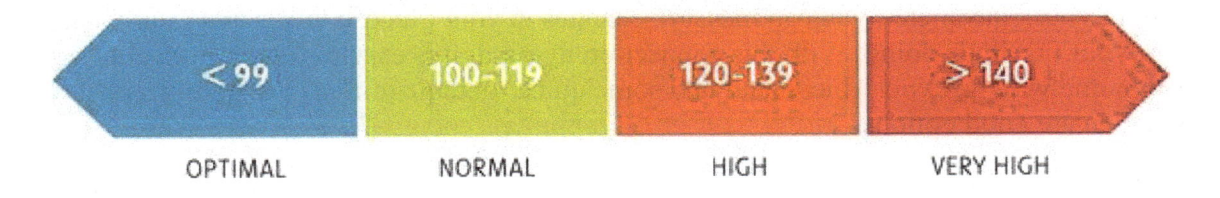

< 99	100-119	120-139	> 140
OPTIMAL	NORMAL	HIGH	VERY HIGH

PRE-BED GLUCOSE (MG/DL)

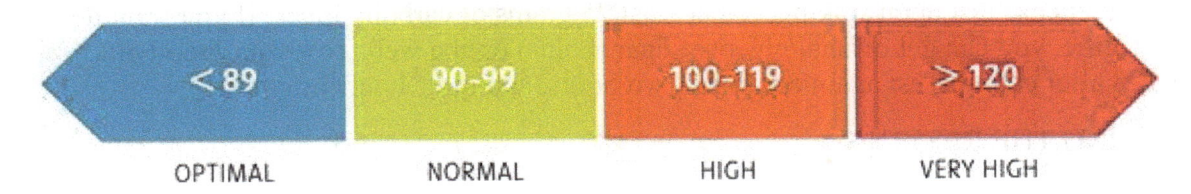

< 89	90-99	100-119	> 120
OPTIMAL	NORMAL	HIGH	VERY HIGH

Category: Food, Hormones

Difficulty: Intermediate

What you need: Glucose monitor and test strips, recording method

Cost: $

INSULIN

ARE MY CELLS STILL LISTENING? AT HOME GLUCOSE SENSITIVITY TEST

WHY THIS TEST
We need to understand how well your cells are listening to insulin. Evidence of your cells not responding well to this hormone means your cells are taxed, and your pancreas is in overdrive. Your cells can heal, but they need time. Where you are now is a result of a lifetime of eating decisions. It will take more than two weeks of good eating to make them healthy again.

WHAT YOU CAN EXPECT TO LEARN

- Observe health of cells in processing glucose.
- Identify early warning signs of insulin resistance.
- Develop a baseline test and monitor over time how cells are healing from good diet decisions.

BACKGROUND

When carbohydrates are broken down in the glucose, the body uses insulin to regulate levels in the blood. With your glucometer, you can measure changes in your glucose levels and infer what kind of work your insulin is doing. With this connection in mind, it is easy to test your insulin sensitivity at home with just your glucometer and some quick (and quantified) fast acting carbs. Potatoes and rice are good options.

Ideally, you want to perform this test every four to six months. For folks who have yet to rein in their carbs and want to start changing their diet, perform this test before and after a diet overhaul. With dedication to a diet, like magic, your cells will return to normal ranges. In the long term, they will thank you by giving you more energy and a trimmer body.

WHAT TO DO

Take a fasting glucose test upon waking. Eat at least 75 grams of carbohydrates. If you want to be more scientific, you can get official glucose sugar (bolus) on the web. Test your blood glucose thirty minutes after eating. Test again one hour, two hours, and three hours after test.

INTERPRETING THE RESULTS

- Fasting blood glucose (mg/dL): < 89
- OGTT post meal (mg/dL after 1 hour): <140
- OGTT post meal (mg/dL after 2 hours): <120
- OGTT post meal (mg/dL after 3 hours): back to baseline

Normal Glucose Chart

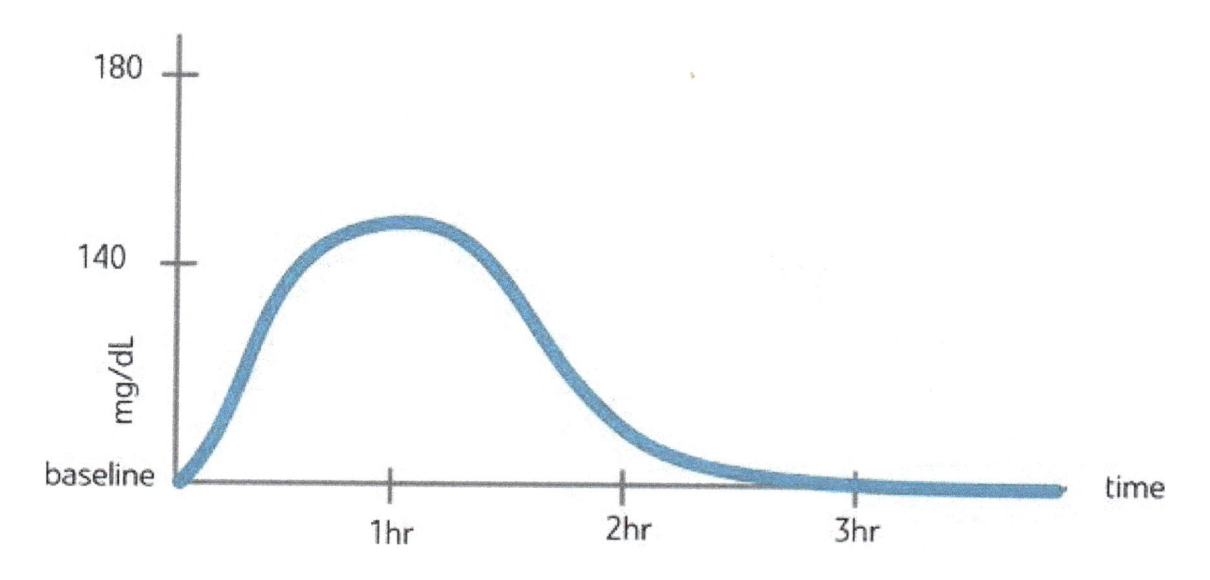

Your glucose levels should rise the first hour. At hour one, levels should be less than 140 mg/dL. At hour three, your glucose levels should have returned near baseline fasting levels. If your chart is normal (didn't rise too high and blood glucose returned to normal after hour three), you're looking good.

If your blood glucose chart looks more like the diagram below, spiking over 140 mg/dL, you are likely to have impaired glucose tolerance and problems brewing. If glucose surges over 200 mg/dL, you need to seek a doctor's help immediately. Glucose is toxic in the blood, so the higher the number, the more damage to your cells. If glucose dips below fasting levels, there is also a problem. Having blood glucose that is too low (hypoglycemia) can be dangerous. This happens when blood glucose drops below 70mg/dL. Finally, if your blood sugar takes longer to normalize, you have just received an invitation to do more digging and to take action.

Abnormal Glucose Chart

Note If you have been living a consistent low-carb diet and are fat adapted, glucose tolerance tests will have skewed results. To account for eating high amounts of carbs your body is not accustomed to, subtract 10mg/dL from 1 and 2 hour readings.

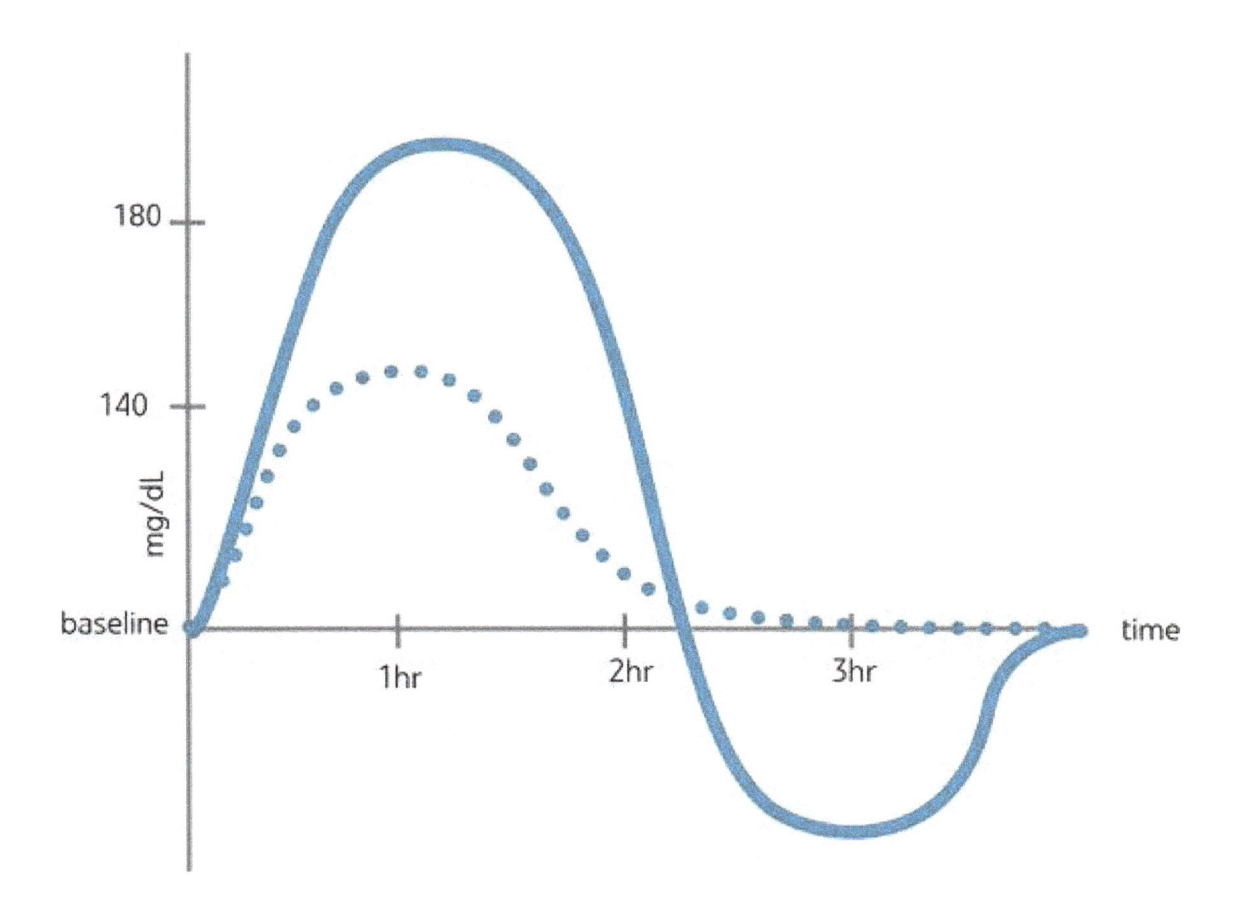

For those with impaired glucose tolerance and have yet to make dietary changes, now is the time. For others on a low carb diet, problems with high blood sugar might be a result of beta-cell reduction, micronutrient deficiency, hormone dysregulation, or autoimmunity. It might be time to seek help to interpret results and collect more information. While we can easily see glucose with at-home tools, other factors are at play including insulin and cortisol. However, these inputs require professional equipment. Seek skilled practitioners to administer tests and help interpret what's going on.

Category: Food, Hormones

Difficulty: Intermediate

What you need: Prescription for blood draw

Cost: $

INSULIN

THE BODY'S GLUCOSE TRACKER: HBA1C

WHY THIS TEST
Your glucose levels are constantly changing throughout the day. While finger-sticking is a great way to get internal snapshots of what is happening at a given moment, it is valuable to know your body's reactions when you aren't looking. Amazingly, your body stores a record of your glucose average in the form of glycated hemoglobin, also known as HbA1c.

WHAT YOU CAN EXPECT TO LEARN

- Blood glucose average over a three-month period.
- Response of body to changes in diet over time.

BACKGROUND
It is difficult to get accurate blood averages. Blood glucose levels fluctuate from minute to minute when you are sleeping, working out, eating, or just daydreaming. One finger stick doesn't tell the whole story. Lucky for us, a metric inside our blood keeps track when we are not looking—a specialized hemoglobin.

Hemoglobin is a transport mechanism inside red blood cells that carries oxygen and carbon dioxide throughout the body. From the lungs, hemoglobin picks up oxygen and travels through the bloodstream to deliver oxygen to tissue. Once delivered, the oxygen is used to burn nutrients to provide energy to power cell activity and function. When oxygen is released, hemoglobin takes the by-product of the cells' work, carbon dioxide, back to the lungs to be dispensed through respiration.

Hemoglobin can transport more than oxygen and carbon dioxide. Glucose sticks to the hemoglobin to make a "glycosylated hemoglobin." This is known as HbA1c. The more glucose in the blood, the more glucose sticks to the hemoglobin.

In a sense this adhesion is the way that hemoglobin keeps track of average glucose levels. Since red blood cells refresh every 8–12 weeks, the HbA1c keeps track over that period of its life. The HbA1c changes slowly, so it is a much better "quantity control" test.

WHAT TO DO

1. Go to your doctor and request a blood draw for HbA1c.
2. Get it specially tested every six months or tack it on anytime you get blood work done.

INTERPRETING THE RESULTS

Translating your HbA1c is easy. Most practitioners recommend this quick equation to convert your HbA1c to your average glucose levels:

$$28.7 \times \text{HBA1C} - 46.7 = \text{AVERAGE GLUCOSE}$$

While a useful marker, HbA1c levels change with the life of cells. Folks with clean diets have healthier cells that live longer and this leads to potentially higher HbA1c levels. Those with poor diets have faster cell turnover with potentially lower HbA1c levels. Use HbA1c in conjunction with the post meal glucose test to get a good picture of what is happening with blood sugar.

HBA1C %: SLOW CELL TURN OVER (LOW CARB)

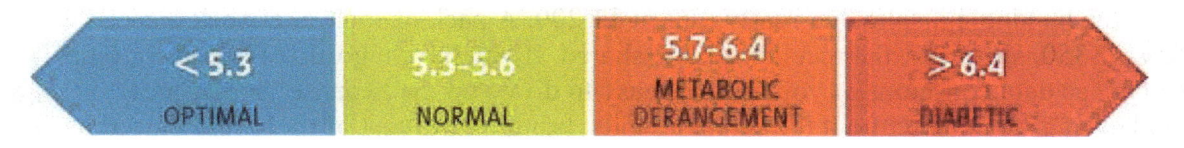

< 5.3	5.3–5.6	5.7–6.4	> 6.4
OPTIMAL	NORMAL	METABOLIC DERANGEMENT	DIABETIC

HBA1C %: FAST CELL TURNOVER (STANDARD AMERICAN DIET)

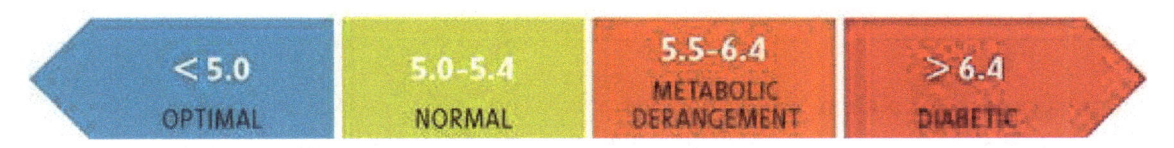

< 5.0	5.0–5.4	5.5–6.4	> 6.4
OPTIMAL	NORMAL	METABOLIC DERANGEMENT	DIABETIC

Category: Food, Hormones

Difficulty: Advanced

What you need: Prescription for device, ability to set up own tests and interpret results

Cost: $$$

INSULIN

LEARNING FROM CONTINUAL GLUCOSE MONITORING: DEXCOM IMPLANT

WHY THIS TEST
A continuous glucose monitor gives you a constant window into what is happening in your body. You will find that surprises abound, and your newly gained understanding will be rich.

WHAT YOU CAN EXPECT TO LEARN

- Identify unexpected culprits of blood sugar spikes.
- Compare the effects of different types of food on your diet.
- Determine best cheat meals that you can tolerant.
- See effects of stress on your glucose levels.
- Test effects of diet soda or other commercial food products.

BACKGROUND

For those extreme self-trackers, another tool is worth mentioning. The DexCom is a continuous glucose monitoring system, which gives you the same amount of data as 288 finger-sticks a day. The DexCom glucose monitor is a wire inserted shallowly into your abdomen, where it remains for a week, held in place with a small patch. The patch sends a wireless signal to a handheld receiver. In addition to live glucose levels, the receiver provides easily readable trend lines that give you a window on how the data is changing in real time.

The DexCom will cost you a pretty penny. The base unit, which includes the device to insert the implant and the handheld display, currently runs at $1,200. A pack of four, one-week disposable patches costs $350. However, the receiver can be shared. If you have a group of friends or gym mates who are as data conscious as you are, it is easy to divvy up the expense. Sometimes doctors and even gyms will rent out the sharable units, bringing the cost of the weekly insert as low as $85. If you seek the large amount of invaluable information you get from the DexCom, it can be well worth the price.

WHAT TO DO

1. Get a prescription for a DexCom device.
2. Before you implant your device, set out a list of experiments and how you plan on doing them.
3. Plan control studies and test runs that change one variable. Implant the device and begin your tests.

Tip: The DexCom is FDA approved to wear on the abdomen. While you cannot feel the guide wire when it is in fat, for those with little fat on their abdomen, the wire can "tickle" muscle, making it noticeable. For those who have little body fat, put the device in a place that has more padding, like your tush.

INTERPRETING THE RESULTS

How to interpret your data depends on the tests you run. Following are samples of tests to run while wearing the DexCom implant.

While most people won't go as far as implanting themselves with a continuous glucose monitor, many have something to learn from the experience. Here are a couple of findings from my own session:

Stress Glucose Connection

The DexCom monitor allows the user to set alerts if blood sugar goes above or below a designated number. I set my device to alert me if my glucose went above 120 mg/dL. Two hours after eating, my device started buzzing. I checked the reading and was astonished. The device read 180mg/dL. How could this be? My food should not have had this result on my blood sugar.

Two hours earlier I had a breakfast of three eggs prepared with one tablespoon of butter from grass-fed cows—a low-glycemic meal. But, my body was responding as though I had just eaten a bowl of sugary cereal. What was going on?

I was suspicious. What was the device telling me? I pricked my finger twice and did glucose tests using a handheld glucometer, just to double check. The high reading was accurate. I immediately did an audit on what I was doing and how I was feeling. I had just entered into what I considered the "zone of productivity" at my work. For me, this feeling seemed like a positive thing; a little bit of adrenaline or stress made me work with a little extra jet fuel. I had always associated this feeling with productivity. But perhaps I had to rethink that—my body had a different interpretation. It seemed like my body was reacting to this stress as a real threat.

It turns out that the stressful feeling that I thought was productive was not doing my body any favors. The stress was stimulating my hormones to call for more glucose to be released into my blood. When I feel that again now, I know that it is time to take a deep breath, relax, and draw my personal jet fuel from another source.

....

Learning:

STRESS INCREASES BLOOD SUGAR. The solution is to take a step back and calm down.

Cheating Smart By Mixing High Carbs Treats With Protein And Fat

We do our best to eat right but at 4:00 PM willpower disappears. Temptation is in your path. You can't say no. Knowing this happens to even the most stalwart of dieters, I wanted to figure out how I could enjoy my treat, while at the same time minimizing the negative effects of the extra carbs on my body.

To do this, I set up a test. I would eat a milk chocolate bar each day, one by itself and one with protein and fat to slow digestion, and I would compare results. The first day, I ate chocolate by itself. This carb binge set my handheld device's warning levels buzzing. My baseline glucose levels were slow to normalize after my chocolate, and for the rest of the day my blood continued to roll up and down all the while trending or "creeping" up. On day two, I ate a candy bar with two hardboiled eggs. The results were better. The protein and fat had dampened the effects of the carbs. A large spike was not seen. I repeated the process again just to verify my results. Eating the candy with something else minimized the ups and downs post candy and allowed my body to recover faster. No glucose creep was seen. It was clear that eating protein and fat with a treat allowed me to avoid big upticks in blood sugar. I was able to avoid the usual post sugar binge ups and downs as well.

Learning:

CHEAT SMART BY INCLUDING SOME PROTEIN OR FAT WITH TREATS.

Skipping meals causes glucose to soar

We get busy and skip breakfast. Sometimes I even think that skipping a meal is doing myself a favor. One morning I woke up at 5:30 AM before leaving town for the day. My blood sugar levels were at 91. In my rush to get out the door, I skipped breakfast. From the moment I woke up, I was moving and busy. No time to stop to eat. At 11:30 AM I finally paid attention to my monitor. It read 125. For my diet this number was high. I pricked my finger and took a test strip to make sure the device was calibrated correctly. It was accurate. Despite my lack of eating that day, my blood sugar was soaring. My body was responding to the lack of food that morning as a stressor and filled my blood with sugar to keep energy up. This was no good. Based on this data, eating a Ding Dong or skipping breakfast had the same effect.

Skipping meals is not always a bad thing. Intermittent fasting can be a regenerative activity for the gut and the body as a whole. However, it's a losing combination to skip meals while continuing to run around living a stressful life or those with poor blood sugar regulation. In the future I will take snacks for those mornings I need to run out the door. When I do fast, I will do so in a cool, collected manner that minimizes stress rather than adding to it.

Learning:

SKIPPING MEALS AND BEING BUSY MAKES BLOOD SUGAR SOAR.

PRACTICE INTERMITTENT FASTING During Periods Of Minimal Stress.

PREPARE MEALS IN ADVANCE that can be taken on the road when time is limited.

Correlation Between Hunger And Blood Sugar Level

In casual conversation the comment, "my blood sugar is low," is used synonymously with "I am hungry." At times after a meal, I feel hungry within an hour. To me it has never made much sense. If I could better understand the message my body was sending, I could better interpret what I should do about it.

During the week I spent wearing my continual glucose monitor, I decided to find out what was really going on with my hunger. I recorded each time I was hungry, and I distinguished between two different types of hunger. One was the subtle compulsion to eat that can be easily ignored. The other was an uncomfortable rumble in the belly. Each time I felt hungry, I made note in my journal of the type of hunger and blood glucose levels.

Looking back at my data, these two forms of hunger were telling me two different things about my body. While the subtle compulsion to eat was associated with lower blood sugar, the uncomfortable rumble in my tummy was not. This meant that sometimes when I was "hungry" my blood sugar was low. I really did need to eat something to stay in range. Other times, my "hunger" was actually due to other factors, such as stomach emptying and contracting, or lack of satiety (leptin/ghrelin), or the snack that I craved was not actually needed. Even though hunger is more complex than a simple blood glucose level, it was useful to know that my findings seemed to have patterns. I observed that the rumble-in-the-tummy hungry feeling happened consistently after drinking diet soda and eating fruit. Going forward, I know that I should really tune into the subtle compulsion that indicates my body's real hunger.

Learning:

BE SENSITIVE TO DIFFERENT SIGNALS FOR HUNGER; the subtle voice is actually more connected to blood sugar levels.

AVOID DIET SODA, even without calories. It makes the body want to eat more.

FRUIT DOES NOT SATISFY HUNGER; reach for a protein or fat-based snack instead.

High carbs, low willpower

This was the test I was looking forward to the most. A carb binge for the sake of science—sign me up! After waking, I sat down to the breakfast of champions, which included glucose pills and a Milky Way—a total of 80 grams of carbs. Happily I chomped away.

Literally two minutes later, my stomach revolted and started cramping as though it had been assaulted. I watched my blood levels rocket up on my glucose handheld monitor with the dreaded double arrow warning sign. Gulp. Two hours later my brain went fuzzy. All I wanted to do was take a nap. I remembered that this feeling was familiar. Before I started eating a paleo diet, I used to feel like this often.

This carb binge was only supposed to be a momentary event. Two hours after I ate my glucose-spiking breakfast, an irresistible craving for more carbs kicked in. It felt like my body was starving and the only thing that could keep it going was sugar. I intended to get right back to eating the way I normally eat to compensate for my morning experiment. But my willpower was nonexistent. My appetite had transformed into an evil monster. Normally full of willpower, I could not resist my body's urge to continue eating poorly—it felt like necessity.

While the life-or-death cravings finally diminished by the evening, it was clear that my body still was much more sensitive to the foods I ate. My glucose levels went through big swings as I ate foods that would normally not cause such a spike.

Learning:

HIGH SUGAR INTAKE CAN LEAD TO DIMINISHED WILL POWER.

BIG SWINGS EARLY IN THE DAY IN BLOOD SUGAR CAUSE GLUCOSE CREEP LATER (EVEN WITH HEALTHY FOODS).

LEARNINGS

As I learned through my experience, continuous glucose level testing with a DexCom can be a powerful tool to change behavior. If you would like to maximize your ability to learn about your body, the findings are worth getting a prescription from a doctor and running your own tests for a week or two. As a result of my own study, I now think twice about skipping meals. I try to address stress when it arises, instead of ignoring it. I also feel confident that the paleo diet I have chosen is the best for me and for my body.

Interpreting Cholesterol and Other Important Blood Work

This section is a practical guide to help you better understand your cholesterol panel. You'll find helpful information, additional important tests that you need to request from your doctor, and trends to monitor. This section provides basic information. It is not meant to be used as a complete understanding of the physiology.

Background

Cholesterol is important. It makes up our cell membranes and serves as a vital structural and functional component for our cells and body. In addition, cholesterol is used to create hormonal messengers. Despite cholesterol's important role as a building block for cells and communications in the body, it is demonized in the public dialogue. Both the lipid hypothesis and the diet-heart hypothesis are responsible for cholesterol's bad rap. The lipid hypothesis claims that high levels of cholesterol in the blood is associated with an increased risk of coronary heart disease. Separately, the diet-heart hypothesis says that dietary fat and dietary cholesterol lead to increases in blood cholesterol and therefore increases in heart disease risk.

At the recommendation of the National Institute of Health, in an effort to be "heart healthy," many gravitate to a low-fat diet to avoid intake of dietary cholesterol. At the same time, doctors run out of ink writing prescriptions for cholesterol-reducing drugs to ward off heart attacks—to the tune of $27 billion a year. The problem? Many who have "normal" ranges of cholesterol still suffer from heart attacks every year. And many with high cholesterol do just fine. While it is true that blood lipids play some role in heart disease, the blame has been placed on the wrong culprit: fat.

DESPITE CHOLESTEROL's IMPORTANT ROLE AS A BUILDING BLOCK FOR CELLS AND COMMUNICATION IN
THE BODY, IT IS DEMONIZED IN THE PUBLIC DIALOGUE.

Attempting to control blood lipids by reducing dietary fat has unexpected domino effects on our body. When we eat dietary fats, our body senses it has enough fats for its construction needs and signals the body's material factories to take a break and use what is available in foods. As a result the body reduces its production of fats for cell repair and growth and reconstitutes fats from food. In contrast when we avoid fats by eating carbs that contain virtually no natural cholesterol, or avoid fat altogether, our body senses a deficiency for the raw materials needed for cell growth and repair and shifts fat production into high gear.

In a world where food was scarce, this process of turning excess carbohydrates into fat (de novo lipogenesis) was advantageous. During a time of plenty, the liver would transform extra carbohydrates into triglycerides and store them as fat for later. When the time of scarcity would come, the body would survive by dipping into fat stores. However, in a hyper-caloric society where food is available all the time, this excess fat storage is less necessary. The result of this low-fat, highly processed, high-sugar diet is high triglycerides and cholesterol. And the "helpful" recommendations cause more harm than good.

Despite cholesterol's important role as a building block for cells and communication in the body, it is demonized in the public dialogue.

Unfortunately many take popular public opinion about cholesterol as ironclad rule. The general population might regularly check and monitor total cholesterol levels, but standard tests don't provide enough information. "Normal" ranges don't indicate optimal health, since they are an average of all patients, many of whom are already sick. For discerning health consumers, you need to educate yourself in order to request the right add-on tests that provide the foundation for meaningful conversations with doctors.

Lipoproteins: The Freight Shuttle for Cell Building

Most are familiar with the term cholesterol. Cholesterol is a type of lipoprotein. Think of lipoproteins as a shuttle. Part protein, part lipid, these shuttles allow materials from the outside of a cell to pass through the cell walls to the inside and deliver needed raw materials. The liver is responsible for making these shuttles. It takes spare parts and recycles materials into useful components (fatty acids, triglycerides, cholesterol, cholesteryl esters, and fat-soluble vitamins.)

Once assembled, these "shuttles" are sent into the bloodstream to distribute raw materials and transport important building blocks for cells of the body. The cholesterol is used to repair and maintain cell membranes, synthesize vitamin D, manufacture bile acids and salts, and synthesize steroid hormones (progestins, glucocorticoids, mineralocorticoids, androgens, and estrogens).

One's risk of developing heart disease is hard to estimate by looking exclusively at LDL, HDL, and total cholesterol. It is not about total number but rather the quality and size of the cholesterol fleet.

When people speak of cholesterol, what is actually being measured is the type and quantity of lipoproteins: very low-density lipoprotein (v-LDL), low-density lipoprotein (LDL), high-density lipoprotein (HDL), and intermediate-density lipoprotein (IDL). But cholesterol is used in discussion because lipoprotein levels are indirectly measured using the cholesterol they transport.

Most doctors or insurance companies look at total cholesterol to determine if you need intervention or are a health risk. But, this method has a problem. It is impossible to estimates one's risk of developing heart disease by looking exclusively at LDL, HDL, and total cholesterol. You need to understand the full picture and look at the various components. It is not about total number but rather the quality of the cholesterol fleet. Some of the shuttles are helpful while others are troublesome. You have to look at the specific types of vehicles (v-LDL, LDL, HDL) to accurately assess what's going on. Lipoproteins can be directly measured by separating them using their differing densities. This, however, is far more time consuming than the indirect measurements that are typically employed.

HDL: The Cleaners

HDL shuttles depart from the liver on a cleanup mission and travel through the bloodstream to collect the junk that is floating around. It also "scrubs" arteries and veins. As it collects these dangerous rogue fats, HDL brings them back to the liver for processing/recycling. Because of its benefits, lots of this HDL cholesterol is desired. You should be worried when you don't have enough of these good shuttles. Ideally, HDL levels should be more than 60mg/dl. People that exercise and eat a smart carb diet can have lots of these good guys.

LDL: The Distributors

While HDL cleans, LDL distributes raw materials. These lipoprotein shuttles transport needed fats, fat-soluble vitamins, cholesterol, and cholesteryl esters throughout the bloodstream to reach the cells of the body. Without the needed supplies, cells can't do their jobs. Most consider LDL as the "bad cholesterol"; however, LDL serves a needed distribution function. Together, HDL and LDL work to clean up the blood and deliver raw materials throughout the body.

In a regular blood lipid panel, the LDL number is a crude gauge for what is actually going on. Instead of actually counting each individual LDL particle, labs calculate this number, using the formula:

LDL cholesterol = total cholesterol – HDL cholesterol – (triglycerides / 5). This formula was developed using certain assumptions, however: HDL must be 40 mg/dl or greater and triglycerides 100 mg/dl or less. Calculations are thrown off when numbers don't fit in this range, which can be misleading for people with metabolic syndrome, diabetes, or genetic conditions.

LDL Particle Size: Why LDL Isn't Always Bad

Not all LDL is created equal. This part of the lipoprotein fleet is differentiated yet again. Among the LDL distributors, the shuttles range in size and density, some are large, buoyant, and fluffy (Pattern A), some are small and dense (Pattern B), and others are intermediate (Pattern A/B). A key to understanding your risk factors is to know what type and concentrations of LDL are in your blood.

Pattern A LDL moves through the blood delivering its goods. The walls of arteries are like nets, and these large, fluffy particles can't get stuck as easily as their smaller and denser counterparts. Some hypothesize that Pattern B particles easily get trapped in microscopic tears of arteries and veins. These little guys can build up, causing plaque and deposits. Gone unchecked, they may break off and float to the heart or the brain, leading to heart attacks or strokes. Others believe that large amounts of Pattern B particles indicate the presence of other problems, such as leptin resistance and down-regulated thyroid function resulting in fewer cholesterol receptors. Either way, it's a smart move to avoid large numbers of Pattern B LDL

Understanding the types of LDL particles in your system will make your cholesterol number useful. There are several tests that can actually count the numbers of lipoproteins in your blood and tell you their makeup. Nuclear Magnetic Resonance (NMR), lipoprotein analysis, and Vertical Auto Profile (VAP) are all examples. However, these tests are relatively new, are not part of standard panels, and may not be covered by insurance. You must specially request them from your doctor or naturopathic practitioner.

To dig even deeper, request an Oxidized Triple Marker Test. This is an innovative cardiovascular disease risk assessment test that measures the number of oxidized small, dense LDL, as well as oxidized Lp(a) (another risk factor for heart disease). Knowing how your particles are oxidized gives a better assessment of your risk for the hardening of arteries (atherosclerosis).

How can we avoid the Pattern B LDL cholesterol problem? One cause of Pattern B LDL is diets with chronically-elevated carbohydrates and insulin. With high insulin, cholesterol production is put into hyper-drive through the upregulation of the enzyme that controls the rate at which cholesterol is made (HMG-Co-a-Reductase). In addition high amounts of trans fats (elaidic acid) and fructose activate Cholesteryl Ester Transfer Protein (CETP) contributing to small, dense LDL particles. Diets with elevated sugar, trans fats, and fructose lead to more "troublemaking" particles.

High carbohydrate diets and chronically-elevated insulin cause high levels of bad Pattern B LDL particles, triglycerides, and low HDL.

Triglycerides: The Fat Makers

Triglycerides are the means by which the body stores fat. When the body has more energy (calories) than needed, it converts the excess into triglycerides— a molecule with three fatty acids linked to glycerol. Triglycerides are transported in the bloodstream by lipoproteins. Fat is normally stored in cells in the form of triglycerides.

The presence of triglycerides was a vital storage adaption when times of famine where guaranteed. Today in a culture of abundance, when calories are always accessible, it is an overused mechanism. Too much of these fat makers in the blood are a bad thing. While it is easy to assume large amounts of fat mean more triglycerides, this is not the case. Unlike sugar, fat is hard to eat in excess. Fat is not addictive, it is satiating, and excess amounts will be purged in the stool.

Those who eat a paleo or low-carb diet can have triglycerides well bellow 100mg/dl. The lower the triglycerides the better. When triglycerides are low, we tend to see strong correlations with high HDL and low Pattern B LDL.

Trends to Watch:

- Triglycerides should go down over time.
- HDL should trend up.
- Total cholesterol to HDL ratio: we want lots of the good HDL. The lower the ratio the better.
- Triglyceride to HDL ratio: ideally this will be close to one or lower.

Trend Watch

Our bodies are dynamic and changing. Cholesterol moves 20-30 points between blood draws. These are natural fluctuations in the body. No need to panic.

Other Lab Work to Monitor

When it comes to blood work, cholesterol is not the only important number you should monitor. Glucose levels and inflammation levels are also keys to getting a good picture of your health. When you get data on your cholesterol levels, also request your markers for glucose and inflammation. Together these markers give a solid picture of what is happening inside your body.

HbA1c: Your Body's Glucose Monitor

Know your blood glucose levels, but constant monitoring isn't for everyone. Luckily, the body keeps track of your average blood glucose. Glucose sticks to a protein in red blood cells, and glucose levels are naturally tracked for about 120 days—the life span of those cells. With an inexpensive blood test, you can have a general read of what is going on with blood glucose over a period of time, called Hemoglobin A1c. Ideal HbA1c levels are less than 5.5 percent. But like many blood tests, it is only an indicator of what is going on in your body. The results have to be interpreted correctly. For instance, if you follow a paleo diet, cells are healthier, and as a result, the cells have a longer life and slower turnover. Over their lifetime they will collect more sugar, so HbA1c levels (average glucose) appear higher than in someone who is eating a Standard American Diet. Their cells turn over much faster—80 days as opposed to 120, so HbA1c levels might be lower, since cells don't live as long. Like many values in medicine, context matters.

C-Reactive Protein: The Inflammation Index

C-reactive protein is a marker for inflammation in your system. This protein binds to the surface of dead and dying cells. When the body is hard at work fighting food, injury, or infection, this marker is elevated. While C-reactive protein is an indicator that a problem exists, it does not tell you what is wrong, so it should be only used as a justification for further testing. Ideally, levels should be less than 1 mg/L.

INTERPRETING CHOLESTEROL AND OTHER IMPORTANT BLOOD WORK

Since total cholesterol and LDL are poor indicators of health, they are not included in this chart.

Instead, focus on particle size, HDL levels, triglycerides, HbA1c, and ratio of Triglycerides/HDL.

HDL CHOLESTEROL MG/DL

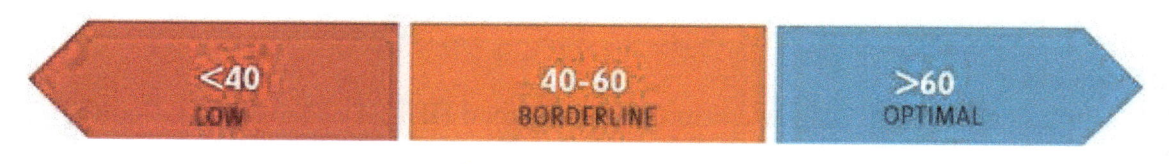

<40 LOW	40-60 BORDERLINE	>60 OPTIMAL

PARTICLE SIZE (NMR)

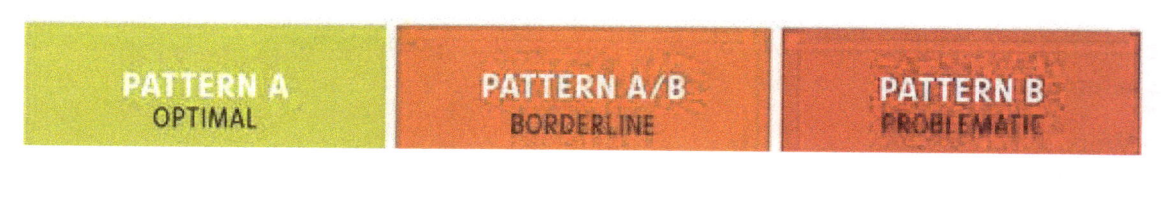

PATTERN A OPTIMAL	PATTERN A/B BORDERLINE	PATTERN B PROBLEMATIC

TRIGLYCERIDES MG/DL

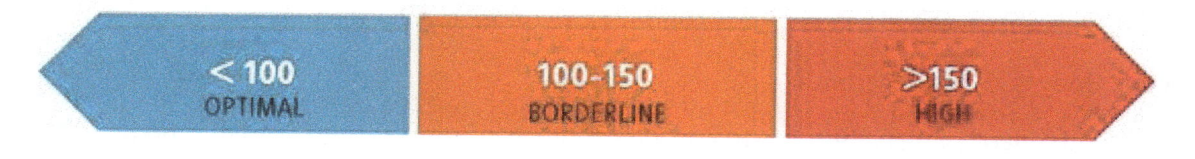

<100 OPTIMAL	100-150 BORDERLINE	>150 HIGH

TRIGLYCERIDE/HDL RATIO

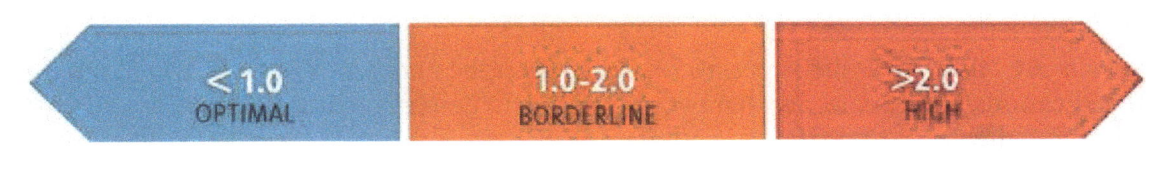

| < 1.0 OPTIMAL | 1.0-2.0 BORDERLINE | >2.0 HIGH |

HBA1C %: SLOW CELL TURN OVER (LOW CARB)

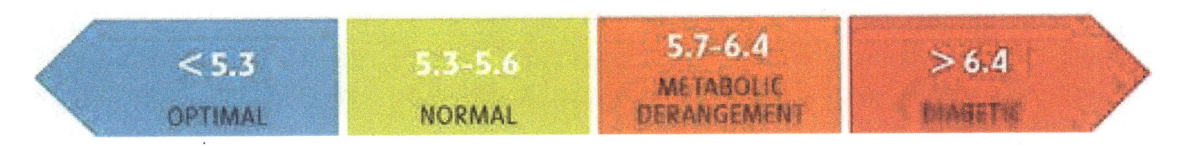

| < 5.3 OPTIMAL | 5.3-5.6 NORMAL | 5.7-6.4 METABOLIC DERANGEMENT | > 6.4 DIABETIC |

HBA1 C %: FAST CELL TURNOVER (STANDARD AMERICAN DIET)

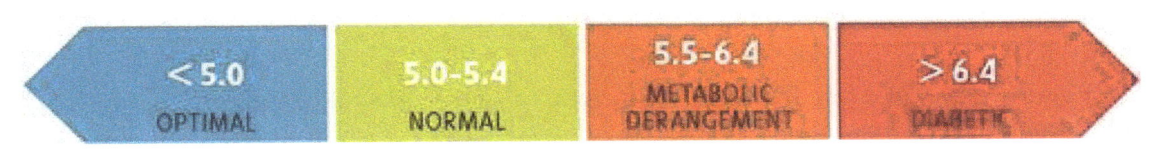

| < 5.0 OPTIMAL | 5.0-5.4 NORMAL | 5.5-6.4 METABOLIC DERANGEMENT | > 6.4 DIABETIC |

C-REACTIVE PROTEIN MG/L

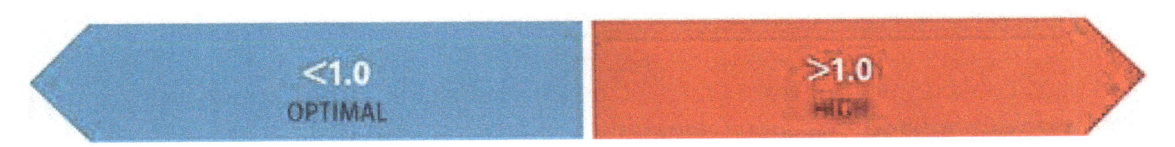

| <1.0 OPTIMAL | >1.0 HIGH |

Design inspired by Thomas Goetz and *Wired Magazine*, "The Blood Test Gets a Makeover."

Category: Food

Difficulty: Intermediate

What you need: Prescription for two cholesterol panels with LDL particle size

Cost: $$

CHOLESTEROL

HOW TO IMPROVE YOUR CHOLESTEROL IN TWO WEEKS WITHOUT DRUGS

WHY THIS TEST

Low-fat products are taking over the supermarket shelves yet the number of people on cholesterol medication continues to rise. Run your own test to determine how cholesterol responds to limiting dietary carbohydrates, not fat.

WHAT YOU CAN EXPECT TO LEARN

- Determine the effects of a low-carb diet on cholesterol.

BACKGROUND

It is easy to conclude that less fat eaten will result in lower cholesterol. But many who follow a low-fat diet don't see their cholesterol numbers drop, making it seem drugs are the only option. Maybe it is time to test a new hypothesis: a diet of limited and quality carbohydrates leads to healthy cholesterol.

WHAT TO DO

1. Assuming you start with a non-paleo diet, take a cholesterol panel including particle size.
2. Eliminate bad carbs: wheat, rice, oats, legumes, and fruit. Add in healthy fats: avocados, olive oil, eggs, butter, nuts, and fatty meats.
3. Record your food intake in a food log. At the end of two weeks, take the same blood panel.
4. Using the information in the interpreting cholesterol section, compare your results to the primary blood work.

SAMPLE MENU

DIET DAY 1
Breakfast: 2–3 eggs cooked in butter from grass-fed cows, ½ cup chopped frozen spinach
Lunch: Cobb salad with nitrate-free bacon, ham, turkey, olives, and balsamic dressing
Snack: Celery with 2 tablespoons of almond butter, 2–3 ounces Paleo Brands beef jerky from grass-fed beef
Dinner: 4–5 ounces steak with a side of baked sweet potato and asparagus

DIET DAY 2
Breakfast: Sweet Potato Frittata
Lunch: Chicken salad
Snack: 2 ounces tuna with 2 tablespoons homemade mayo on cucumber slices
Dinner: Pork chop with steamed broccoli, butter, and side salad with balsamic vinaigrette

DIET DAY 3
Breakfast: 2–3 eggs cooked in grass-fed butter, ½ cup grain-free granola with coconut milk
Lunch: Hamburger (no bun) wrapped in lettuce, grilled onions, and side salad
Snack: Leftover frittata from the day before
Dinner: 3–4 ounces salmon, grilled squash, cauliflower rice with butter

DIET DAY 4
Breakfast: 2–3 eggs cooked in butter from grass-fed cows, 1 breakfast sausage
Lunch: Leftover salmon from dinner with veggies
Snack: Justin's Almond Butter squeeze packet
Dinner: Halibut with Citrus and Sweet Potato

What you can expect to see: HDL should rise. LDL should go from Pattern B (bad guys) to Pattern A (good guys). Triglycerides should go down.

Category: Food

Difficulty: Advanced

What you need: Ketone blood tester or ketone strips

Cost: $$

CHOLESTEROL

LEARNING FROM A FAT-FILLED DIET: EXPERIMENTS IN KETOSIS

WHY THIS TEST
While talk abounds about the low-carb diet, the no-carb (very low-carb) diet is worth experimenting with. Ketosis affects dopamine receptors in the brain and is neuroprotective (protective of brain neurons). This will give you a chance to chart your diet, and its effects.

WHAT YOU CAN EXPECT TO LEARN

- How your body and brain react to no carbohydrates in the diet
- The effect of high fat on basic cholesterol, particle size, and triglycerides.

NOTE:
Consult your doctor before going into ketosis. This is not for pregnant women—stick to a smart carb diet instead. Ketosis is not to be confused with Ketoacidosis, a dangerous condition encountered by type 1 diabetics who experience uncontrolled ketone production due to lack of insulin.

BACKGROUND
When we consume fewer carbohydrates than required for basic functioning—usually less than 50 grams of carbohydrates per day—the body turns to other sources for energy: proteins and fats. When the body breaks down fats, by-product fuel molecules, ketones, are created. When these ketones accumulate in the blood at high levels, it is known as ketosis. This state, when controlled, can offer health benefits that are typically lacking in our carb-rich diets.

Ketogenic diets range from moderate to therapeutic. For example, low-carbohydrate diets include periods of ketone production and therefore are moderately ketogenic. When carbohydrate levels are severely limited, insulin and glucose are curbed. Ketones increase in the blood until they become the main fuel source. Therapeutic levels of ketosis are used to treat many brain disorders, such as epilepsy and multiple sclerosis. Three main types of ketones are produced in the blood: beta-hydroxybutyrate, acetoacetate, and acetate.

The human body was designed to function well in the presence of ketones. Ketones are used in many of the metabolic pathways where carbs exist. For many systems in the body, ketones and carbs are used interchangeably. Ketones are a preferred fuel source for the brain. This is why low-carb diets help with clear mental functioning and high-carb diets leave you with a feeling of mental fogginess. But, more importantly, ketones protect neurons from oxidation and oxidative stress, making them less susceptible to degenerative brain diseases such as Alzheimer's. They also help regulate dopamine (the happy makers), and they have been hypothesized to help regulate depression. For decades, ketosis has been recommended by doctors as a last resort to fight persistent seizures. Beyond the brain, other cells in the body also respond well to ketones. One type of ketone, beta-hydroxybutyrate, is a super fuel. It increases energy while decreasing oxygen consumption, making cells more efficient at doing their job.

Testing the level of ketones in your body can be done through a variety of means. The most convenient and least expensive method is to use over-the-counter urine tests that detect the presence of ketones. However, these ketone strips are not the most reliable method. Ketones in your urine are evacuated as a waste product, so they don't always correlate to the amount of ketones in your blood. And, as your body adapts to the diet, your tissues adapt to using ketones as fuel, becoming more efficient at making and using the right amounts of ketones. As a result, excess ketones are not as present in urine, making the ketone strips less reliable.

KETONES ARE A PREFERRED FUEL SOURCE FOR THE BRAIN. THIS MAY BE WHY LOW-CARB DIETS HELP WITH CLEAR MENTAL FUNCTION AND HIGH-CARB DIETS LEAVE YOU IN A FOG.

Testing can also be done with ketone monitors. They are more accurate but more expensive. Ketone monitors work the same way as glucometers, requiring a finger prick and test strips. The amount of ketones in your blood depends on the level of ketosis your body is in.

KETOSIS RANGES
measured in Millimolars

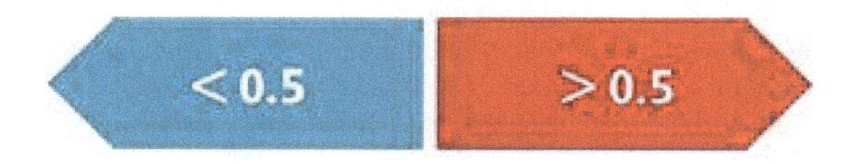

< 0.5   > 0.5

Many of the benefits of a ketogenic diet can be achieved through maintaining low to moderate levels of ketones in the blood. For those who are using ketosis as a tool to fight depression, cancer, or neurodegenerative disease, the opportunity to halt the progression of the disease or minimize the use of medication may be worth the experiment.

WHAT TO DO

To set up the experiment, identify what you are testing. Are you testing the effects of a high-fat, low-carb diet on your cholesterol? Or are you testing the effects of ketosis on your happiness? Before starting, get a blood panel taken, including LDL, HDL, triglycerides, and particle size.

Make changes to your diet. Seek the following ratio:

1 GRAM COMBINED CARBOHYDRATES AND PROTEIN : 4 GRAMS FAT

To calculate your daily macronutrients, start by calculating your protein requirement. Amount of daily protein is based on your body weight. To maintain muscle mass you will need .36 grams of protein per pound of body weight. The basic formula is:

YOUR WEIGHT X .36 = GRAMS OF PROTEIN YOU SHOULD AIM TO EAT EACH DAY

For example, if you weigh 150 pounds, your protein intake should be 150 lbs x .36 g = 54 grams of protein a day. If you weigh 200 pounds, then aim for 72 grams of protein a day.

For many who are already on a low-carb diet, these protein values will seem low. However, proteins can also turn into glucose. We need to be careful not to overeat this macronutrient to maintain the ketogenic response to fat as our primary fuel. The ideal scenario is to have just enough protein to maintain muscle but not more. Use your ketone test monitor to follow how your body reacts to varying amounts of protein in your diet. Determine your ideal protein intake to allow yourself to maintain the desired level of ketosis. Tweak your diet to find your ideal measures.

A low-carbohydrate diet shifts your body (specifically your kidneys) from retaining salt to excreting it. If you find yourself thirsty or experiencing headaches, your body is suffering from mild dehydration due to this loss of salt. Supplement your ketosis diet with salty bone broth or, if necessary, the less natural bouillon cubes to ward off side effects.

Seek to consume up to 1–3 tablespoons of Medium Chain Triglycerides (MCTs) a day, preferably in the morning to get your ketone metabolism going. MCTs are found naturally in fats like coconut oil. Isolated versions can be purchased as supplements at health food stores. Unlike other fats, MCTs burn more like carbohydrates—the body utilizes them immediately. MCTs are also the most ketogenic fats, meaning they are most readily transformed into ketones by the body. Because they are turned to fuel so quickly, they can be used as a pick-me-up to help boost ketones in the blood when your energy is waning. A warning: MCT oil is a laxative, build up gradually.

If you are experimenting with this diet for extended periods of time, connect with a doctor or dietician who can work with you. When fats become 80–90 percent of your source of calories, specialists often recommend supplementing your diet with a multivitamin, fish oil/cod liver oil, and selenium.

Record how you feel, your mood, and what you ate. Take blood ketone tests five times a day—upon waking, two hours after meals, and before bed. When your numbers are below the suggested range, cut back on proteins. After one month, take your basic blood panel again.

INTERPRETING THE RESULTS

Compare starting values and ending values.

How did you feel? What has happened to your weight? How did your caloric consumption change? How did your HDL, triglycerides, and LDL particles change? Did you lose weight and inches off your waistline? How did you feel? The case studies below are designed to help you get a sense of the possibilities for a ketosis diet.

This diet has a major downside: it eliminates sweet potatoes! Rest assured, though; those smart carbs will be extra delicious when you cycle back into your regular diet.

Case Study #1: Ketosis and Athletes

Brian is an extreme athlete. He loves to be in the pool, on his bike, or in the gym. He regularly spends three hours a day rotating between swimming, cycling, and weight lifting. Over the years he has put his fitness to the test competing in open-water, long-distance swims, triathlons, and cycling races.

Disciplined in his training and diet, Brian was looking for a new variable to tweak in preparation for an upcoming bike century. He began to focus on increasing power output by losing weight, rather than by increasing training. If he lost fat, he reasoned, his ratio of power to body weight would increase. Based on the "calories in, calories out" argument, he could either eat less or work out more. Neither were good options to maintain his high level of performance. Instead, Brian experimented with another tool: ketosis.

Brian was diligent about recording his information. When he started, he weighed 195 pounds with 20 percent body fat, as measured by a DEXA scan. He took a lipid panel with particle size and a VO2 max test. He tested his blood several times a day to monitor ketone bodies and carefully adjusted protein levels to maintain high ketogenic ranges.

He changed his diet from a medium-carb, high-protein diet to high fat, low carbs, and protein. Brian used the Ketosis formula and self-testing to arrive at his ideal ratios. Here are his daily micronutrient breakdowns as a proportion of his calories:

Daily Macro Nutrient Breakdown Before and After Ketogenic Diet

	BEFORE	**AFTER**
CARBS	35%	4%
PROTEIN	25%	8%
FAT	40%	90%
CALORIES	3,500	4,500
ACTIVITY (Hours)	3	3

His friends looked on in horror as he consumed a small bowl of olive oil, a steak with extra butter, and then finished off with the fat discarded from his friend's meat. But the diet did not stop there. While fellow endurance athletes would train with sports gels, Brian packed blocks of cream cheese to chow away on long rides. When he tried to explain that he was attempting to lose weight, his friends would roll their eyes. They politely warned him about the dangers of high-fat diets and cholesterol.

Looking at Brian's numbers, conventional wisdom would expect that over three months his 30 percent increase in calories and his 105 percent increase in fat consumption would lead to skyrocketing cholesterol, but this was far from the case.

Eating a high-fat, no-carb diet helped Brian lose 25 pounds on an already slim frame. Fat melted off. But that is not all. While his cholesterol saw an overall increase, a closer look showed the nuance behind the numbers. The thirty-point rise in cholesterol was driven mainly by large jumps in HDL (good cholesterol) and large buoyant particles of LDL. So, despite the rise in total cholesterol, it was the good cholesterol that changed most dramatically, not the heart-stopping small LDL particles. The results didn't end there. His aerobic efficiency also improved, while his body became less dependent on glucose. This means that his cells became more efficient at burning fat, an important advantage for long-distance athletes who require refueling.

The final result was increased cell efficiency, increased good cholesterol, and less body fat. As Brian explains, ketosis was worth it, and his anaerobic activity was the only thing that suffered.

CONVENTIONAL WISDOM WOULD EXPECT A 30 PERCENT INCREASE IN CALORIES AND 105 PERCENT INCREASE IN FAT CONSUMPTION WOULD LEAD TO SKYROCKETING CHOLESTEROL, BUT THIS WAS FAR FROM THE CASE.

A Look at Cholesterol Before and After Ketogenic Diet

	BEFORE	AFTER
BODY WEIGHT (LBS)	195	170
BODY FAT (%)	20	7.5
WAIST MEASUREMENT (Inches)	35	31.5
FOOD (K/Cal)	3500	4500
CHOLESTEROL TOTAL (Standard)	**144**	**144**
LDL	113	59
HDL	31	85
TRIGLYCERIDES	154	81
TRIGLYCERIDES/HDL RATIO	4.97	0.95
INSULIN SENSITIVITY (HOMA-IR)	1.38	>0.48
INSULIN LEVELS BEFORE (mU/L)	6	>2
INSULIN LEVELS 2 HOURS AFTER	36	16
GLUCOSE LEVELS BEFORE (mg/dL)	93	97
GLUCOSE LEVELS 2 HOURS AFTER	108	83
CHOLESTEROL TOTAL (VAP)	**141**	**145**
HDL TOTAL	58	67
HDL 2 (large, more protective)	17	27
HDL 3 (small, less protective)	41	42
LDL TOTAL	**61**	**77**
LDL 1+2 (large buoyant)	24	25
LDL 3+4 (Small dense)	37	26
REMNANT LIPOPROTEIN (LDL + VLDL3)	22	26

Case Study #2: Ketosis and Depression

John was born with an unfortunate genetic trait—depression. He became aware of a problem in high school. He remembered feeling down for "no reason" for months at a time. His sadness and anxiety continued to become more and more pronounced throughout the years, and in his twenties obsessive-compulsive behaviors emerged.

Depression, anxiety, and obsessive behaviors were quite a combination of symptoms. John worked with doctors at Stanford University to help come up with a cocktail of medications that would help alleviate the symptoms. The right combination of drugs was hard to find. Although drugs helped, they came with side effects.

With the negative side effects, countless visits to doctors, therapy sessions, and the high daily expense for medications, John got fed up and sought other solutions. While reading the paper one Sunday, John came across an article about the use of ketosis to keep seizures under control. He reasoned, "if ketosis helped stabilize the brain against seizures, it might be a tool to help fight depression." Fascinated, he wanted to learn more. He eagerly read research papers and blogs.

While little research had been done on the effects of ketosis to fight depression and anxiety, it was clear that ketosis helped the brain. John shared his findings with his doctor. While public literature only hypothesized about depression and anxiety, he ran his own experiment to see what results he could experience. He tracked what he ate and his anxiety for two months, moving toward a therapeutic level of ketosis.

For years John had been an on-again, off-again smart carb eater. He typically had periods of strict compliance, followed by sugar binges. He felt that tracking himself at this baseline over a month would give him enough time to observe these behaviors and their effects.

One morning, his office had piping hot bagels. John could not resist the smells of a bakery wafting through the halls. Two hours after eating those carbs, his anxiety set in. The anxiety was so bad that he contemplated coming home from work. This was his first clue. High-starch foods appeared to make his symptoms worsen.

Looking at the baseline data from his month of regular eating, it was clear that he was the least compliant with his low-carb diet choices when he felt the worst. In his daily life, cookies had become a type of self-medication. However, through his experimentation, he could see that the momentary improvement to his feelings from eating a bag of cookies was followed by days of negative ripple effects on his mood. As he continued to explore, again and again, he began to see a pattern. High-sugar, high-starch foods made him feel worse.

Next, he began to transition to a ketogenic diet, at the same time working with his doctor to reduce medications. What happened? A high-fat diet lowered some of the background anxiety and depression. Ultimately, while symptoms did not totally disappear, the big swings in his mood were eliminated. John describes himself in his new lifestyle as "much more steady." He is hopeful that with this change he can work with his doctor to wean himself off medications. John is optimistic and realistic about the results. While he is not afraid to use medications "if things get rough," he is pleased to be able to have a lifestyle tool to be able to manage his issues on an ongoing basis. He currently is on less medication with fewer side effects.

Category: Inflammation, Activity

Difficulty: Advanced

What you need: Prescription for a blood test

Cost: $

INFLAMMATION

IS MY BODY INFLAMED? C-REACTIVE PROTEIN

WHY THIS TEST

Chronic inflammation is an underlying cause of excess weight. It lays the foundation for heart disease and other chronic illness later in life. We can see the physical effects of acute inflammation, but it is more difficult to see what is going on inside the body. Data on inflammation levels in the blood can give us this valuable information.

What you can expect to learn

- Identify levels of inflammation in the body.

BACKGROUND
C-reactive protein is found in the blood and rises in response to inflammation in the body. This protein binds to the surface of dead and dying cells. Monitoring this protein is a great way to understand what is happening. Are your cells in working order? Or are some sick and dying? Sick cells cause inflammation that taxes the roadways of your veins and arteries.

Unfortunately, C-reactive protein only identifies the presence of inflammation. It does not tell you what that inflammation is from. Since high levels of inflammation require more sleuthing to understand, doctors may choose to limit how they use it for diagnostic purposes. However, the tinkerer can learn a lot from this simple test. Change one variable at a time and see what happens, gathering clues about possible causes. As an added bonus, this test will show you the effects of your healthy eating effort. Take the test before and after changes in your diet to see your progress.

WHAT TO DO

1. Get a prescription from your doctor.
2. Take the test when healthy to get an accurate baseline reading. Illness or injury throws off the number. Also, hard workouts cause a breakdown of cells, leading to higher levels of inflammation. To avoid skewing your results, get blood drawn before you workout.

INTERPRETING THE RESULTS

The ideal level of C-reactive protein is less than 1 mg/L, but the number will skyrocket when you are sick or hurt. Are your numbers high even though you are healthy? Eliminate grains, dairy, and legumes. Incorporate anti-inflammatory foods such as fish. Test again after two weeks. Numbers still high? Is your over-exercising breaking down your body so much it can no longer repair itself? Adjust the intensity of your physical activity. Take the test again. If your numbers are still high, seek a health care professional to work with you to get to the bottom of the problem.

Category: Food, Inflammation

Difficulty: Intermediate

What you need: Discipline, body awareness

Cost: Free

INFLAMMATION

IDENTIFYING PROBLEM FOODS: INTOLERANCE/ALLERGY STUDY

WHY THIS TEST
Some foods, whether part of a paleo diet or not, cause irritation in our system. At the extreme, these foods cause allergies. For most, they cause only low-grade, annoying symptoms, including digestive discomfort, gas, bloating, or pain. Even if reactions are not severe, consistent low-grade exposure to foods our body doesn't like can be a cause of chronic inflammation.

WHAT YOU CAN EXPECT TO LEARN

- Interpret cues from your body to identify problem-causing foods.
- Determine foods that cause allergies or low-grade stress on your digestive system.
- Identify foods to avoid.

BACKGROUND
Grains and legumes that ravage the gut are not the only dietary culprit of inflammation. While some of us might do fine with dairy, others can't tolerate it. A strict paleo diet can eliminate many of the low-grade allergens in food, but as with any diet, you lose access to many foods you enjoy. As you adjust and try to find a balance between strict paleo and a livable middle ground, allergies and discomfort can come back with a vengeance.

If we understand the foods that our body doesn't like, we can avoid them. While doctors offer blood tests to determine allergies, results are not always reliable. The most effective test is to clean up your diet by omitting foods that are potential allergens. Once your system is clear and reset, you introduce foods back in, one at a time. When the body doesn't like something, you will notice. You will have gas, bloating, or headaches. Your body is trying to speak to you through these symptoms. You need to pay attention in order to adjust your response to your body's needs. While this does take weeks of discipline, the outcome can be insightful.

WHAT TO DO

1. Commit to diet for a four- to six-week period. The first seven to twelve days is a detox period, containing only foods that are unlikely to be allergens.
2. Eat only these foods: organic turkey, lamb, squash, peaches, cauliflower, cabbage, cranberries, sweet potatoes, lettuce, olive oil, filtered water, pears. This means no coffee, tea, alcohol, or other beverages except water.
3. At the end of the detox period, begin to introduce foods back into your diet. Eat the same new food at each meal for one to two days. If you feel a reaction to a food, discontinue it from your diet and wait for symptoms to clear before introducing the next food. Common allergens to introduce one at a time include: dairy; citrus; shellfish; seafood; beef; refined sugar; peanuts; eggs; potatoes; corn; rice; nuts; tomatoes; soy products; bananas; and caffeine products, including chocolate, tea, coffee, and soda.

As you eat these new foods, record how your body responds. How do you feel? What do you notice? Is your body speaking to you?

INTERPRETING THE RESULTS

Pay attention to all kinds of symptoms during the trial.

SYMPTOMS MAY INCLUDE abdominal pain, cramping, diarrhea, or excess gas. If you experience these symptoms you can consider yourself intolerant. Pains and discomfort in digestion are not the only symptoms to experience.

OTHER SYMPTOMS CAN INCLUDE:

Skin reactions—itching, burning, hives, red spots, sweating, etc.

Ear, nose, and throat—sneezing, runny nose, sore or dry throat, hoarseness, ringing in the ears, dizziness

Respiratory—wheezing, mucous formation, shortness of breath

Cardiovascular—increased heart rate or pounding heart, flushing, tingling, faintness

Gastrointestinal—increased salivation, canker sores, indigestion, bloating, stomachache, heartburn, constipation, pain, diarrhea, gas

Genitourinary—frequent, urgent or painful urination, inability to control bladder, itching, discharge, pain, water retention

Musculoskeletal—fatigue, weakness, pain, swelling, stiffness of joints, backache

Nervous system—headache, migraine, drowsiness, inability to concentrate, depression, irritability, restlessness, hyperactivity, dizziness, numbness, tremors

At the end of the trial, you will have a safe food list and a list of foods to avoid. Foods you are allergic to cause damage to your body; eliminating food your body does not tolerate gives your body time to heal. If the food is one you can't live without, try reintegrating it six months later. But be honest with yourself; if your body rejects something, you have to trust it. If you are intolerant of many random-seeming foods, this might be a sign of leaky gut, autoimmune conditions, SIBO, or a gut pathogen. A gut-healing protocol may be in order.

Category: Hormones

Difficulty: Intermediate

What you need: Prescription for cortisol test

Cost: $$

CORTISOL

IS MY BODY STRESSED? DAILY CORTISOL PATTERN

WHY THIS TEST
Cortisol is the stress hormone that circulates in your body. Acute cortisol elevation from time to time is expected as you go through challenges in life. Chronic cortisol, however, can cause stress on our bodies and make us store fat, especially in our midsection, where abdominal fat cells are particularly sensitive to this hormone.

WHAT YOU CAN EXPECT TO LEARN

- Determine if you are experiencing chronic stress.

BACKGROUND
Beyond its function as a fight-or-flight stress hormone, cortisol gets our bodies moving in the morning. A healthy person's cortisol starts out highest in the morning, and then gradually declines throughout the day, reaching its lowest levels three or four hours after sleep. For someone with a stressful lifestyle, cortisol follows a similar pattern, but at much higher levels.

We can test our cortisol levels to understand how our bodies are dealing with the stress of everyday life. Testing can be done either through a blood panel in a lab, or at home by collecting saliva samples throughout the day and sending them to a lab by mail. While a blood test gives you a single snapshot, saliva tests over the course of a day will provide a view into your body's trends. Testing can be done through your doctor or with test kits ordered from the web. Prices vary widely, so compare before ordering.

Cortisol

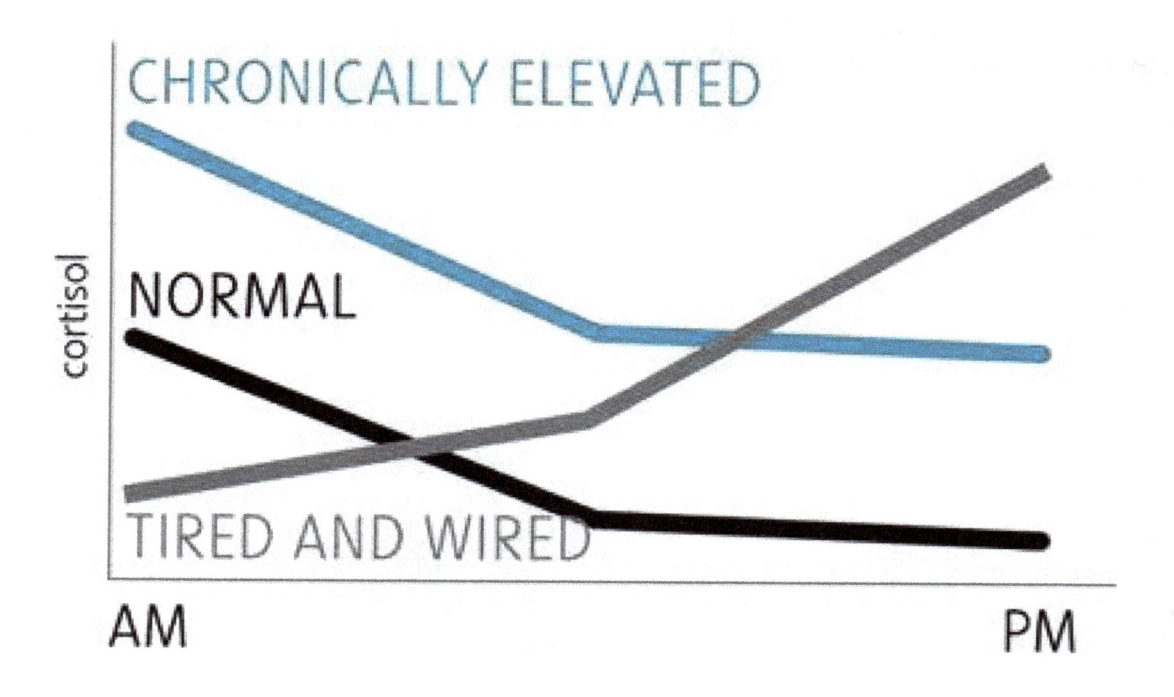

WHAT TO DO

1. Get a prescription for a cortisol test from your doctor.
2. Take the test over the course of a day.

INTERPRETING THE RESULTS

Normal cortisol should start out high in the morning. By afternoon, levels should taper and reach low levels at bedtime. Chronically high levels of cortisol are often well above normal levels and can indicate problems. Other abnormal cortisol patterns start out low and end high at the end of the day.

De-stressing is not just self-indulgent New Age mumbo jumbo; controlling your base levels of cortisol, through stress management, is important to your health. Here are some tips to help manage those base levels:

- Say no to drama
- Minimize exposure to stressful people
- Eat regularly
- Limit uppers, like caffeine, to the morning when cortisol levels are naturally high
- Practice sitting still
- Breathe deeply
- Take a walk
- Do yoga

Category: Hormones, Activity

Difficulty: Intermediate

What you need: Prescription for pre- and post-stressor cortisol test

Cost: $$

CORTISOL

CHOOSING THE ACTIVITY THAT IS RIGHT FOR MY BODY: CORTISOL RESPONSE TO EXERCISE

WHY THIS TEST

Just as the insulin factories grow weary from overwork, so do the cortisol factories. This is called adrenal fatigue or adrenal insufficiency. When our adrenal factories are not working, we are run down and don't see gains in our performance. Understanding how your adrenal glands are functioning can help you choose the activity that will give your body what it needs—stimulation to get stronger or rest to recuperate.

WHAT YOU CAN EXPECT TO LEARN

- Identify how adrenal glands are responding to acute stressors.
- Determine if specific exercises are causing more harm to your body than good.
- Choose activities that are right for your body now.
- Identify reasons for feeling run-down and not seeing gains in performance.

BACKGROUND

Acute stressors—isolated instances of stress—can be caused by brief confrontations, challenges at the office, blowups at home, or even exercise. We cannot control most of the acute stressors the world throws our way. We can, however, control the stress we give ourselves from exercise. The right kind of exercise builds muscle tone, increases insulin sensitivity, lowers blood pressure, strengthens bones, and lowers stress, making you feel good. The wrong kind of exercise adds to already high levels of stress, and the physical benefits of this type of exercise come at a cost.

What are the right and wrong types of exercise? Like many questions in health, the answer depends on you and your unique physiology. While lifting hard and heavy is great for some, yoga is better for others. What is good for each of us depends on baseline stress levels in our lives, as well as how often, how hard, and how long you have trained.

YOUR BODY WANTS TO BE HEALTHY. LISTEN TO IT AND ACT SMARTLY.

If you train hard consistently, always pushing for maximum effort or until failure for years, your cortisol factories might be running on fumes. You have probably noticed that your performance and fitness levels have hit a wall. In order to see more progress, your adrenal glands have to be rested and work within their limits.

How you feel and perform can be a great starting point to determine if your body is overstressed by the exercise you are inflicting on it. If you are depressed, lethargic, have no desire to work out, have slow recovery times, find your performance at a plateau, or, for women, experience irregular menstruation, these are signs your body is fatigued and your cortisol factories may be overworked.

Testing cortisol before and after a stressor, like exercise, gives you a view of how your adrenal glands, the cortisol factories, are keeping up. While some doctors may charge you a hefty $600 to run lab work, you can use online services for around $200. If you are an athlete who is consistently pushing to the limit, this is a good investment. For instance, Bio Health Laboratory (www.biodia.com) offers an exercise tolerance test and skilled doctors to help you interpret results.

WHAT TO DO

1. Plan a workout between 4:00 and 8:00 PM, when cortisol levels should be low.
2. Test yourself before activity.
3. Perform your workout. When finished, do another test. Send in your results for processing.

Normal Cortisol Chart

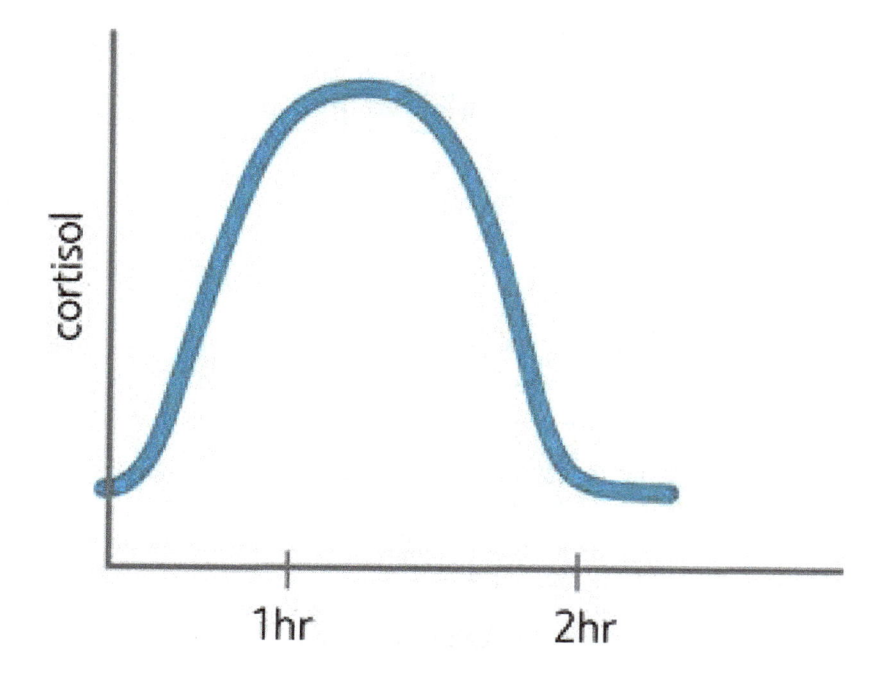

INTERPRETING THE RESULTS

A normal graph should look like the one at the left. The starting value is your baseline. After exercise, cortisol rises then drops one hour after exercise, returning to baseline two hours after exercise. If cortisol levels drop below your baseline levels, this means your exercise decreased stress. Win!

Abnormal Cortisol Charts

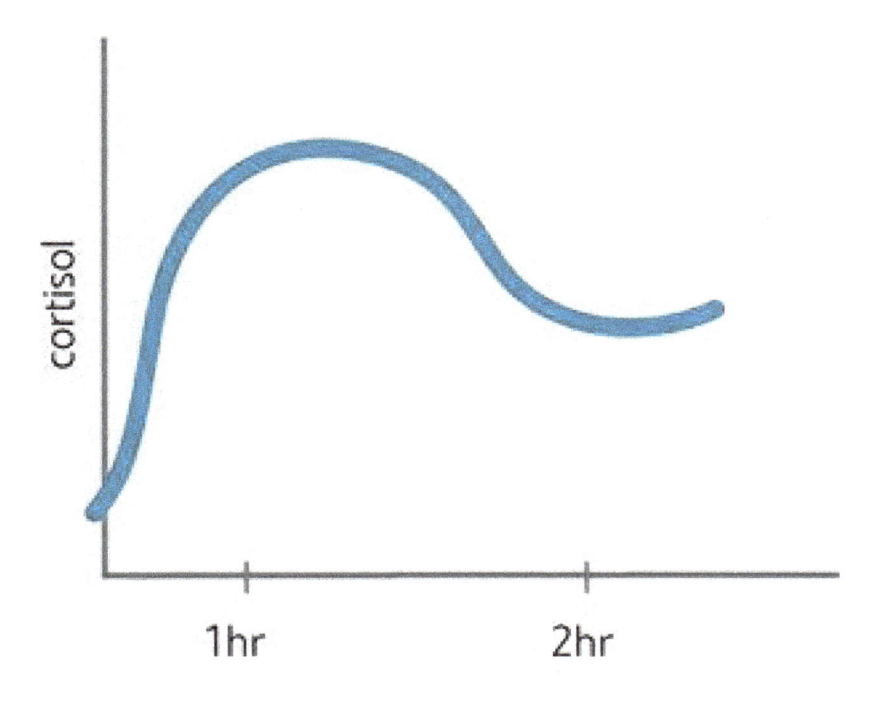

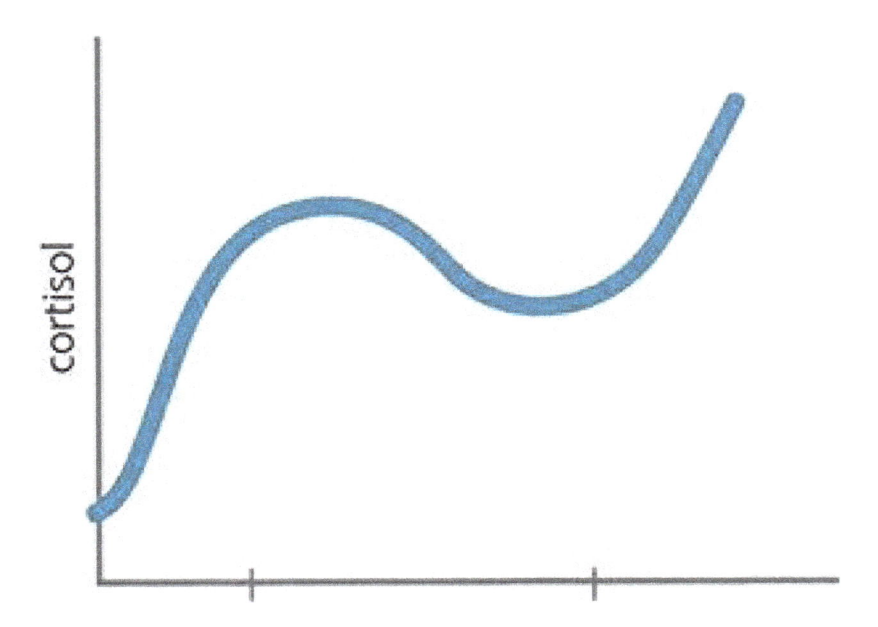

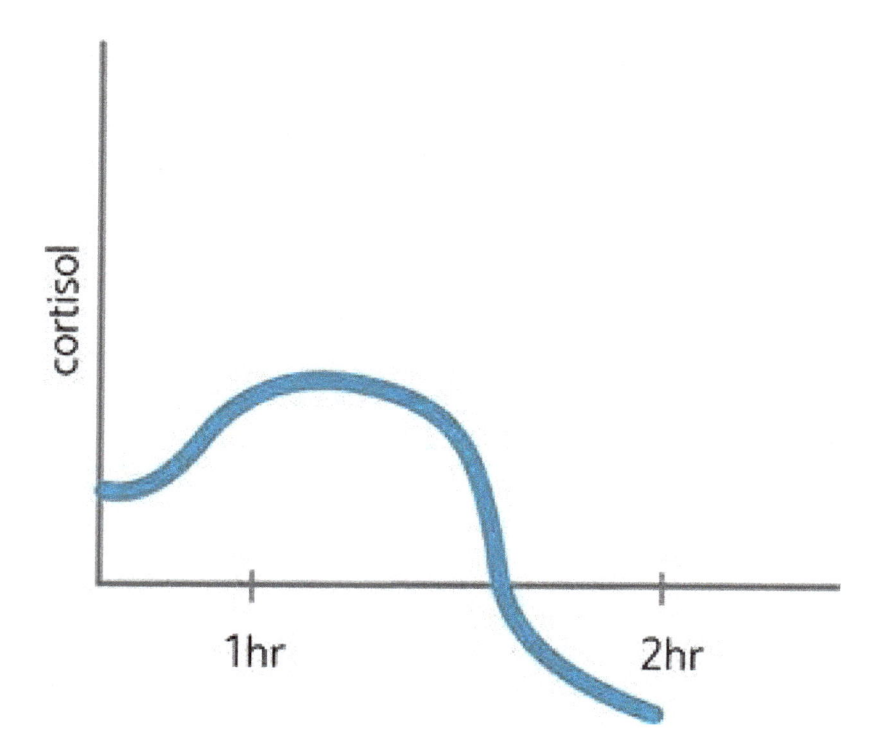

If your graph is different than the normal arc above, then your exercise caused you more stress or the cortisol factories are fatigued. Your body can react abnormally after a stressor in three different ways:

1. Cortisol can rise without a return to baseline. This response indicates that the type of exercise you are doing is adding stress instead of decreasing it.
2. Cortisol can rise and then continue to rise. Here the body is responding to the stress as if danger is imminent and it anticipates more stress.
3. Cortisol levels raise only a little and then dip well below baseline. This indicates late-stage adrenal fatigue. The body is so tired that it no longer can muster the ability to compensate for the stresses demanded of it.

IF YOUR ADRENAL GLANDS ARE STRESSED FROM CONSTANT HARD EXERCISE, LET THE BODY REST AND REPAIR SO IT CAN COME BACK EVEN STRONGER.

If you respond to an exercise stressor abnormally, take note and consider backing off. Your body was programmed to function in cycles of hard work and rest. Rest gives the body a chance to repair, recover, and grow. We are not designed for constant activity or stress. Exercise is hard work and we want to make sure that all that effort is doing our bodies good, not damaging us. Understanding where you are in the cycle is an important part of smart training.

If your adrenal glands are taxed, give your intensive exercise a rest for a couple of weeks or months. Choose instead an activity that doesn't stress your body, such as walking, yoga, or swimming. This lifestyle change does not have to last forever. You can get back to your long bike rides, runs, and heavy lifting soon enough. The self-imposed rest period will bolster your physiology, give your body a chance to repair itself, and come back even stronger. For those who have made intense exercise a part of daily life, this transition can be hard. Be kind to yourself. Taking a break is not laziness—resting is smart training. Ease slowly into your training regimen and make note of how you feel. If you start to experience adrenal fatigue symptoms again, seek help from a doctor or other practitioner to explore other possible causes and treatments.

Category: Food, Hormones, Inflammation, Activity

Difficulty: Easy

What you need: Access to a blood draw lab

Cost: $$$

FOOD, HORMONES AND ACTIVITY

GET ON TOP OF YOUR HEALTH: THE GRAND DADDY OF BLOOD WORK; WELLNESSFX

WHY THIS TEST
WellnessFx provides at least 50 diagnostics at a single go. Since they are outside of the healthcare system, costs are kept low (less than paying by cash through a doctor). You don't have to ask for a prescription, and you have skilled practitioners to help interpret trends across systems of the body. Doctors coach you in addressing the roots of problems through smart lifestyle recommendations (instead of just drugs). All this and easy-to-understand, visualized data online.

WHAT YOU CAN EXPECT TO LEARN

- Uncover hidden problems area.
- Systems approach towards the body.
- Effect of lifestyle and dietary changes on blood values.
- Guidance to interpreting results.
- Actionable lifestyle changes.

BACKGROUND
The body is a complex system. While most blood tests give a snap shot of a particular marker, it can be hard to get a holistic sense of what is going on. Some doctors may not have the time to sleuth. Patients without an immediate problem can be a lower priority.

Valuable tools are emerging while at the same time cost is dropping. San Francisco-based WellnessFx runs a comprehensive panel of over 50 diagnostics ranging from metabolic panels, including thyroid, female and male sex hormones, cardiac, liver, and kidney functions to many vitamins and minerals. Unlike many other testing companies, their goal is not to sell vitamins or drugs. Instead, they aim to provide insight and let the data encourage behavior change. Follow up blood work is done after several months to show the results of your efforts.

While costs are currently expensive, up to $1,500, they are coming down. For those interested in making this type of data a regular part of their health care, WellnessFX also has a monthly fee that provides member blood work twice a year with follow-up.

WHAT TO DO
Individuals sign up online and are issued a prescription for a blood draw. Once analyzed, easy-to-read and fun-to-engage data is shared online.

INTERPRETING RESULTS
When the results are available, phone consultation with knowledgeable doctors will help you sleuth through your personal data and find the insights unique to you. Together you map out a plan for lifestyle changes to help address problem areas. When medications or supplements are recommended, physicians will work with you across systems of the body so that patients can be on the minimum effective dose in combination with lifestyle and dietary changes.

VALUABLE TOOLS ARE EMERGING WHILE AT THE SAME TIME COST IS DROPPING.

Case Study

James is a CrossFit coach who works out regularly and takes nutrition seriously. He plays careful attention to his diet and eats lots of protein to maintain muscles while limiting carbohydrates.

Even though he is in tip-top shape, he recently took the WellnessFx panel and was surprised by the results. While most athletes would expect high levels of testosterone, his was low. The precursors of testosterone dehydroepiandrosterone (DHEA) mirrored the results. Low testosterone is a key hormone in muscle growth and repair and fat metabolism. Without enough, one cannot reap the full rewards of a workout. Clearly, even in good health, he had something to improve upon.

Collaborating with WellnessFx doctors, James went through his patterns to identify causes for this marker. First, they discussed increasing weight lifting to increase testosterone. However, James was already participating in heavy weights 3-4 times per week. Next, they explored sleep. Since poor sleep can decrease testosterone, the WellnessFx team discussed lifestyle. It was clear that James takes his sleep seriously and makes sure to get more than adequate rest. Finally, they discussed diet. James shared his diligence to eat protein and limit carbs. Problem solved. Limited fat constrained the formation of testosterone. He upped healthy dietary fat, saw changes in his testosterone, and broke through a performance plateau.

Food	Hormones INSULIN	Hormones CORTISOL	Inflammation	Activity	
Eat sweet potatoes to increase nutrition density and fill the body up with good carbohydrates	Eat sweet potatoes to help cells become more sensitive to insulin	Eat sweet potatoes to limit excess stress response from food	Replace egregious carbs with sweet potatoes to limit and fight inflammation in the body		No Rx needed ↑
Limit fruit and fructose in diet	Sleep more to increase insulin sensitivity	Limit stress		Incorporate activity into your daily life	
Limit carbs	Eat low carb foods that do not spike glucose and insulin, avoiding a cortisol kick			Fuel activity with sweet potatoes for good energy while avoiding fructose	
Count carbohydrates		Sleep in a blacked-out room to reduce stress			
Eat paleo: meats, vegetables, nuts, seeds, little starch, little fruit, no sugar	Eat fat and protein to limit food affects on blood sugar		Eat paleo to avoid grains that cause inflammation	Eat paleo to maximize performance and recovery	
Determine your optimal level of carbohydrates using symptom guide	Test Hb1Ac	Take a daily cortisol level test	Test C-Reactive protein to measure baseline inflammation markers in the body	Fuel smartly during your post-workout fueling window	
	Test bedtime glucose		Perform elimination test to identify food allergens	Pre-and post-stressor tests to determine if activity has healthy effect on cortisol levels	
	Test glucose after meals			Test adrenal function to detect fatigue	
	Glucose tolerance test				Rx and testing needed ↓

CHAPTER TAKEAWAY

Some of us are just now getting our carbs and diet under control. Others are further along the journey—tweaking glucose, testing cortisol, and cycling in and out of intense exercise. Where we are on the path doesn't matter as long as we are moving toward health. Once we start testing and see what's going on firsthand, we gain motivation from feeling healthier, while simultaneously seeing our results improve.

The chart on the left is organized by the equation for optimal health and can help you understand each component that can be changed, tested, and monitored. Columns are organized from easiest lifestyle changes to those that require a doctor's order. As you move down, more tests are added based on complexity—the first done with over-the-counter products and ending with tests that need orders from doctors. The chart below is a quick guide to glucose testing.

A quick guide to the glucose numbers

Test	Optimal	Normal	Metabolic Derangement	Diabetic
Fasting Glucose (mg/dL)	<89	90-99	100–119	>120
Pre-bed Glucose (mg/dL)	<89	90-99	100-119	>120
Glucose 1 hour after eating (mg/dL)	<119	120-139	140-199	>200
Glucose 2 hours after eating (mg/dL)	<99	100-119	120–139	>140
Glucose tolerance test (mg/dL after 1 hour)	<99	120-139	140-199	>200
Glucose tolerance test (mg/dL after 2 hour)	<99	100-119	120-140	>140
HbA1c (%)	<5.3	5.4-5.7	5.7–6.4	>6.4

Part IV

THE SWEETNESS OF THE SWEET POTATO

GETTING TO KNOW THE VERSATILITY OF THIS NUTRITIONALLY-PACKED FOOD

CHAPTER 8

SWEET POTATO BASICS

—

INCORPORATING THIS POWER FOOD INTO YOUR EVERYDAY DIET

We thrive when we eat quality foods designed by nature and appropriate for our unique biology. The right foods give us balanced hormones + low inflammation + properly fueled activity. Now it is time for the delicious task of figuring out how to connect our optimal lifestyle to the sweet potato that will help keep us healthy.

Getting to Know This Superfood

Many foods high on health are short on taste. Not the sweet potato. This root is sweet and delicious and, if prepared correctly, even indulgent. While the sweet potato will bolster your health, it will also have power over your taste buds.

The tasty recipes that follow illustrate how versatile sweet potatoes can be. As main dishes, sides, or even desserts, sweet potatoes can be easily incorporated into delicious meals and on-the-go snacks. Let these recipes inspire you. Eliminating bad carbs (wheat, rice, corn, sugar) in a diet and eating more smart carbs like sweet potatoes should be a delicious, nutritious pleasure, not a lifestyle sacrifice.

It's time to get to know this underappreciated little root and give it a deserved place in our diets throughout the year.

WHAT DO YOU DO WITH A SWEET POTATO?

BE ADVENTUROUS.

Sweet potatoes can be prepared and used in many different ways: grate-it, cube-it, slice-it, mash-it, cut-it, wedge-it, or stuff-it. You can't go wrong with sweet potatoes!

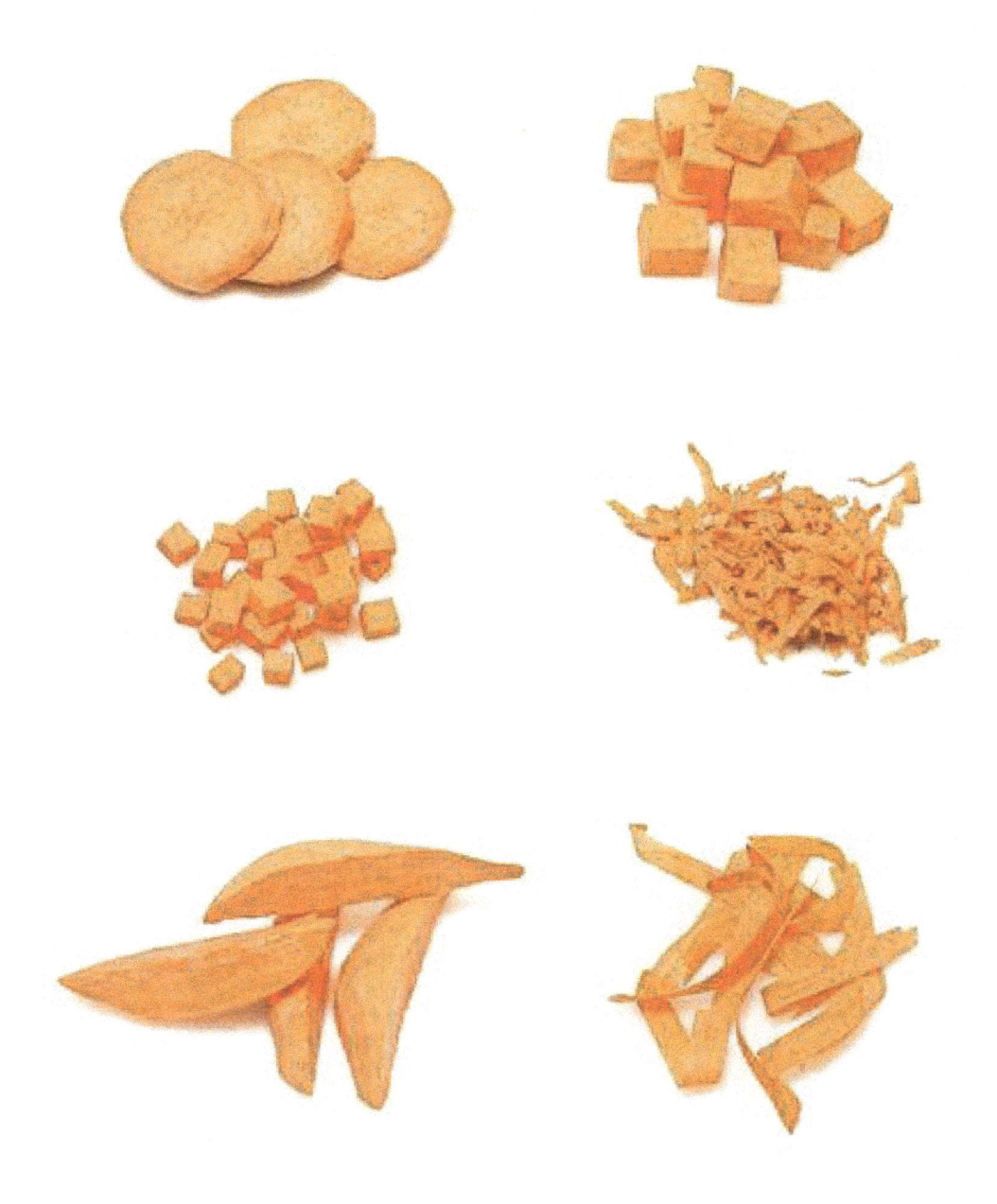

TYPES OF SWEET POTATOES

Hundreds of sweet potato varieties exist with a diversity of skin and flesh colors and levels of sweetness. Skin color ranges from beige or earthy brown to reddish or copper tones to deep purple. Flesh colors range from white or yellow to light or deep orange to purple. Most supermarkets carry only a few varieties. Here are the most commonly seen sweet potatoes in the United States—each has its own unique qualities.

Sweet Potato Classic

Mention the sweet potato and this is the variety that comes to mind. It has a light beige skin and a white-yellow flesh. This variety is drier and less sweet than the bright-orange flesh varieties and is firmer when cooked. The Hannah and O'Henry are common sweet potato varieties.

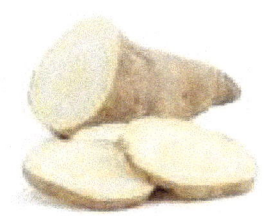

Yams

Yams have a copper, red-toned or dark red skin and bright orange flesh. These are the culprits of confusion. Sweeter and moister than their white-fleshed brethren, they are the mainstay at the American Thanksgiving table. They shine without all the marshmallows, brown sugar, and maple syrup. When baked, yams produce a moist, sweet, syrupy flesh. Most of the recipes in the following section call for yams. Their bright orange flesh reveals a high presence of beta-carotene or vitamin A. The Garnet, Jewel, and Beauregard are common yam varieties.

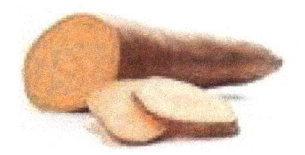

Okinawa Sweet Potato

Open these unassuming, brown-skinned roots and you will find a rich, intense purple on the inside. Purple pigment is due to anthocyanins—the same goodness that makes blueberries blue. Yes, that's right: you can have all the healthy benefits of blueberries (important antioxidant and anti-inflammatory properties) without the fructose. Some might mistake these snacks for cake or other sweets. Don't believe me? Just look at the impulse buy area next to the checkout register at 7/11 stores in Okinawa. Okinawa sweet potatoes win the space that is typically occupied by candy bars in the United States. You can even see Okinawans in flip-flops chasing sweet potato carts through the streets for these caramelized treats. Seriously, they are that good.

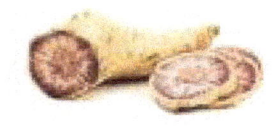

Japanese Sweet Potato or Satsumaimo

Meet the Satsumaimo, the super sweet potato from Japan that turns into coveted caramelized goodness. This gem is red on the outside and a light yellow on the inside. When baked, the Satsumaimo caramelizes into a decadent treat—clean carbs equivalent to cupid's arrow to the heart.

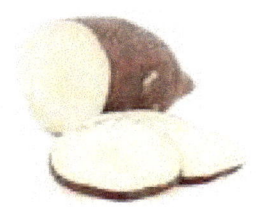

Where to Buy the Lesser-Known Varieties of Sweet Potatoes

Most grocers carry only a couple of varieties of sweet potatoes or yams. With some effort, however, you can experience the diverse range of tastes that the sweet potato has to offer. Check out your Asian markets for the Okinawa and Japanese varieties. Also, you can explore farmers' markets for more heirloom varieties. Be adventurous. The rewards, like the sweet potatoes themselves, are sweet and healthy.

PRACTICAL GUIDE: KITCHEN TIPS FOR THE SWEET POTATO LOVER

Eating right gives you the health and vitality of a superstar. No self-respecting superstar wants to use all that energy working in the kitchen. It is easy to get to the goodness in sweet potatoes with a couple of timesaving shortcuts.

THE FREEZER IS YOUR FRIEND. No tool in the kitchen makes the sweet potato more accessible than the freezer. In addition to their taste and nutritional awesomeness, sweet potatoes freeze like a dream. On those days when you feel the urge to tap your inner Julia Child, stock up. Bake a batch of sweet potatoes, so good nutrition need not be a chore. Using the tools in your kitchen effectively allows you to beat the time conundrum and get the most gain with minimal effort.

BATCH PREP FOR CONVENIENCE TO MINIMIZE EFFORT. Baking sweet potatoes in the oven takes about an hour, depending on size, and optimizes their sweetness. Once you have a store of baked sweet potatoes, incorporating them into your diet is easy. After baking a batch, mash them (see Basic Sweet Potato Prep section). Place the mash in silicone cupcake trays and wrap tightly. Freeze. Each week, remove a few from the freezer tray and store them in an airtight container. Grab one for a quick, on-the-go snack, or use the mash when called for in recipes. If you want to be really clever, measure how much each tray cup holds so you know how many to defrost for upcoming recipes.

GET TO KNOW YOUR OVEN. Today's oven is a cook's best friend. Learn the settings. Many models allow you to pop something in the oven and set cook start and stop times. You can have piping hot sweet potatoes to fill your post-exercise glycemic deficit as soon as you arrive home from work or finish your workout.

PLAN THE RIGHT FUEL FOR THE JOB. If you are running, you are not going to be using utensils to eat. For quick power in your back pocket, try steaming a small sweet potato. It will keep a firm form, minimizing the squish factor. Also, during long exercise periods, taste buds can become more finicky. Steaming avoids the enhancement of sugar, which, for some, becomes unpalatable during extended exercise. Running an ultra marathon? Think of making a sweet potato gel substitute in a squeeze container.

LAZY IS FINE, BUT BE SMART—CANNED SWEET POTATOES. Canned organic sweet potatoes are an easy substitute for recipes calling for baked sweet potato purée. Check the label to be sure that no sugars have been added.

LEARN THE STORE-BOUGHT OPTIONS. Tasty varieties of sweet potato chips, oven fries, and wedges abound. Go for brands that are baked, not fried, and check for hidden ingredients (sugar or gluten).

"THE DELICATE FLAVOR OF THE SWEET POTATO IS LOST IF IT IS NOT COOKED PROPERLY... A SWEET POTATO COOKED QUICKLY IS NOT WELL COOKED. TIME IS AN ESSENTIAL ELEMENT. TWENTY MINUTES MAY SERVE TO BAKE A SWEET POTATO SO THAT A HUNGRY MANY CAN EAT IT, BUT IF THE FLAVOR IS AN OBJECT, IT SHOULD BE KEPT IN THE OVEN FOR AN HOUR." GEORGE WASHINGTON CARVER, 1936

HOW TO BUY SWEET POTATOES:

- Look for sweet potatoes that are small to medium in size.
- Select firm sweet potatoes with even skin coloration, and with no cracks, bruises, or soft spots. Any blemishes on the surface quickly spread to the inside, ruining the whole sweet potato.
- Avoid sweet potatoes with any signs of decay.
- Avoid any with a white, stringy "beard," a sign that the potato is over mature.

STORING AND HANDLING SWEET POTATOES IN YOUR KITCHEN:

- Store sweet potatoes in a cool, dry place, away from the stove.
- Remove sweet potatoes from packing plastics. If bags are necessary, place in a paper bag with ventilation holes poked into it.
- Do not store uncooked whole sweet potatoes in the refrigerator. It alters their taste and makes them form a hard core.
- Handle sweet potatoes carefully to prevent bruising.

- When cutting sweet potatoes, always use a stainless steel knife to avoid color change. A carbon blade causes the sweet potato to darken.
- For the best flavor and freshness, use your sweet potatoes within a week or two after purchase.

BASIC SWEET POTATO PREP:

Sweet potatoes lend themselves to a variety of preparation methods. Each brings out different characteristics and flavors. Sweet potatoes are more nutritious if cooked with the skin on. Begin your preparation by washing and scrubbing under running water.

BAKING Baking sweet potatoes releases their natural sugars, bringing out the tasty goodness and caramelizing them to perfection. Preheat oven to 400 degrees. Prick with fork and place sweet potatoes on a cookie sheet covered with aluminum foil. Bake until tender when pierced with a knife, approximately 50–60 minutes for small to medium (do not wrap in aluminum foil, they will steam not bake). If left to sit overnight, the sugars will caramelize even more. To save time and energy, bake several at a time. Cool and wrap individually in foil and store in freezer bag to freeze or refrigerate.

MICROWAVING Microwaving is quick and easy. The downside is they won't have the sweet, syrup flavor of oven-baked sweet potatoes. Pierce with a fork or knife, place on a paper towel, and microwave on high until tender, approximately 4–5 minutes, depending on the size. Turn over halfway through cooking. Remove and wrap in aluminum foil to rest for at least 5 minutes.

STEAMING Steamed sweet potatoes are less sweet but they retain their shape if taken on a run or eaten as a snack later. Boil 1 cup water in a steamer. Place whole, unpeeled sweet potatoes in steam basket and cover. Steam until tender when pierced with a fork, around 15 minutes, depending on the size of sweet potatoes. Leaving the peel intact prevents excessive loss of precious nutrients and "locks" in its natural sweetness.

BOILING Boiling sweet potatoes is another quick prep method. Place whole sweet potatoes, unpeeled, in boiling water and boil until tender when pierced with a fork, about 30 minutes depending on size. Drain, cool, and peel.

SAUTÉING Sautéing is quick, but it also brings out the natural sweet flavor.

If not organic, remove the outer skin of the sweet potato with a potato peeler. Slice, dice, or cube the sweet potato into the desired shape. In a nonstick pan, heat oil or butter on medium-low heat. Sauté the sweet potato until tender. Depending on the shape and thickness, sautéing takes only a few minutes.

RAW Grated raw sweet potatoes in salads add nutrition and crunch. Scrub under running water. If not organic, remove the outer skin with a potato peeler and grate. If serving raw sweet potatoes as an appetizer or eating as a snack, to avoid discoloration, cut or slice into desired shape (sticks or rounds) and place in ice water or in a plastic bag with ice water for 10 minutes. Drain and serve.

GRILLING Grill on an open or closed grill over medium-hot coals, or for gas grill on medium-high, until sweet potatoes begin to brown and are tender when pierced with a skewer, about 10 to 20 minutes depending upon size.

Recipe Measurement Guide

Sweet potatoes vary in sizes. For the following recipes:

- A medium-size sweet potato, approximately 16 ounces, measures approximately two cups mashed, cubed, sliced, or grated.
- A small-size sweet potato, approximately 8 ounces, measures approximately one cup mashed, cubed, sliced, or grated.

INGREDIENTS IN THESE RECIPES:

Note: Quality matters. Dishes burst with flavor when fresh ingredients are used. Seek out farmers' markets, specialty stores and other vendors that have the freshest offerings.

Here is a bit of background on the foods used in these recipes:

Meat and fish: To maximize nutrition, choose grass-fed meats and wild, line-caught fish. Just like us, animals and fish are healthier when they have eaten according to their natural diets in the wild.

Vegetables: Seek out vegetables grown locally and in season to maximize nutrients. Fresh food bursts with flavor—it's nature's green light. If food falls flat, chances are its nutrition is waning, and you should buy fresher next time. Organic-grown produce is best, as it is raised with organic fertilizer and free of pesticides.

Nuts and seeds: Nuts and seeds are a staple for any diet based on nature's nutrition. Full of energy and nutrients, these are great garnishes for dishes and easy ways to add texture. Purchase nuts and seeds raw and roast them yourself to avoid hidden sugars found in processed nuts.

Some starch: The sweet potato is the smart carb food. Packed with nutrition, fiber-filled and dense, the sweet potato's long list of health benefits speaks for itself, in stark contrast to wheat-based products, which can be harmful to our bodies.

Little fruit: Filled with fructose, fruit should have a limited role in a diet. Skip fruit snacks and instead use fruit to add flavor and variety to dishes. Avoid drinking fruit juice. By being judicious about how and when fruit is consumed, you can take advantage of its delicious taste without loading up on its liver-filling sugars.

Sweeteners: While refined sugar is a no-no, raw honey and pure maple syrup can be used occasionally. In the days of our primal ancestors, these goodies were seasonal and hard to find. They should be used sparingly.

Milk: Dairy is not part of a traditional paleo diet. The few recipes here with dairy use raw milk and cream rather than highly processed variants. The pasteurization process kills many healthy nutrients.

Butter: Seek out high-quality butter from cows or goats that are grass fed, including brands such as Kerry Gold from Ireland. Butter from grass-fed animals has superior nutrition, including higher levels of Omega-3 fatty acids. That's the good stuff.

Gluten-free flour: One recipe uses gluten-free flour. While far from an ancestral food, this is a good alternative to wheat for a cheat day, once in a while. C4C flour, for instance, can be substituted cup for cup to regular flour. Even if we aspire to a paleo diet, having an alternative to the most egregious diet offender—wheat—can provide the treat to satisfy cravings.

Kosher salt: Kosher salts contain no preservatives or added iodine. The salt has larger, irregular grains that add a bit of crunch when added at the last minute to foods. For salad dressings and baking, ground sea salt or table salt is used as it dissolves more quickly.

Fats/oils: Pantries filled with good fats help you feel full and satisfied. For salad dressings use high-quality, extra-virgin olive oil. Nuts such as almonds, walnuts, hazelnuts, and macadamias can be used for added nutritional fats. For oil in dishes that require medium to medium-high heat, use coconut oil, unprocessed palm oil, or lard. Unlike olive oil, these fats are stable at high temperatures. Purge your cupboards of canola, safflower, and fake shortenings. These options are extracted from grains and, unfortunately, a staple of the American kitchen.

Some might look at these recipes and object that they are not all paleo. The paleo diet is a general guideline. It is up to you to interpret what works for your body's unique needs. Some might tolerate dairy, others might not. Some do well with sweet potatoes every day, some do not. With the formula for optimal health and the tests in the self-monitoring section, you now have the tools to make your own rules.

CHAPTER TAKEAWAY

Now that you know the different types of sweet potatoes and how to prepare them, dive into the recipes and have some fun. Mix, remix, and don't be afraid to add or substitute sweet potatoes in any of your own favorite recipes!

Sweet potatoes are one of the most nutritionally-packed foods. They should be the delicious cornerstone for a diet that supports optimal health year-round. The sweet potato isn't a silver bullet that will guarantee your health. Build your lifestyle around the pillars of good food, low stress, low inflammation, and healthy activity. With this holistic approach, sweet potatoes will give you the nutrition you need, help you keep your hormones and inflammation at healthy levels, and provide fuel for exercise that keeps your body lean, all in one of nature's most delicious forms. This is how you can harness sweet potato power to help you thrive!

CHAPTER 9

PRIMAL RECIPES FOR A MODERN WORLD

FROM BREAKFAST TO PERFORMANCE ENHANCERS: ALWAYS A SPOT ON THE TABLE FOR THE SWEET POTATO.

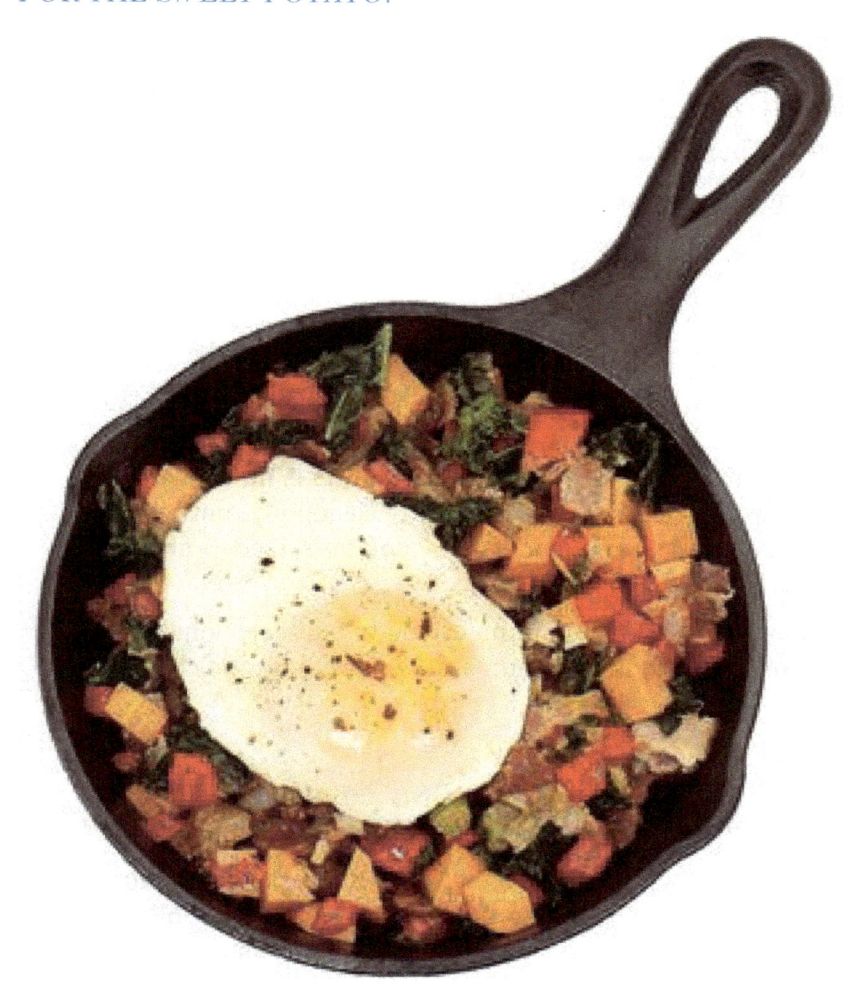

Morning Hash With Sweet Potato

This recipe can go head-to-head with any traditional American breakfast. The vibrant flavors will make your palate dance. Make the hash ahead of time. When ready to eat, heat and crack the eggs on top. Morning Hash is a filling treat after coming home from a big workout on a weekend morning.

Serves 4

> 8 strips of bacon, nitrate free, cut into ½-inch pieces
> (kitchen scissors make it fast and easy)

1 Tbsp extra-virgin olive oil

1 medium onion, chopped

2 cloves garlic, minced

1 large red bell pepper, chopped coarsely

1 small yam, peeled and cut into ½-inch cubes, about 1 cup

1 bunch kale, tough stems removed, chopped

1 tsp fresh thyme, chopped

Kosher salt and freshly ground pepper to taste

....

1. In a large frying pan over medium heat, cook bacon until crisp. Transfer bacon to a paper towel to remove fat. Clean pan of excess fat. Add oil to pan and heat to medium.

2. Add onions and bell pepper. Sauté, stirring 1–2 minutes until onion is translucent. Lower heat and add garlic and yams. Cover and cook, stirring occasionally, until yams are tender and start to brown, about 5 minutes. Add kale and cook until tender, about 5 minutes. Stir in thyme and bacon. Salt and pepper to taste.

3. Crack four eggs over the mixture. Cover. After 2 minutes add two tablespoons of water to the pan. Replace cover and cook another minute or two until eggs are cooked to desired doneness.

Braised Apples and Sweet Potato in Spiced Honey over Grainless Granola

Breakfast sets the course of food choices for the rest of the day. Set up success with a nutritious, healthy, hearty start. Make a batch of this satisfying stew so you have something to pull out of the refrigerator in the morning. You can put it on top of grainless granola, or you can simply heat, eat, and go. The braised apples and sweet potatoes also make a delicious side to pork.

Serves 4

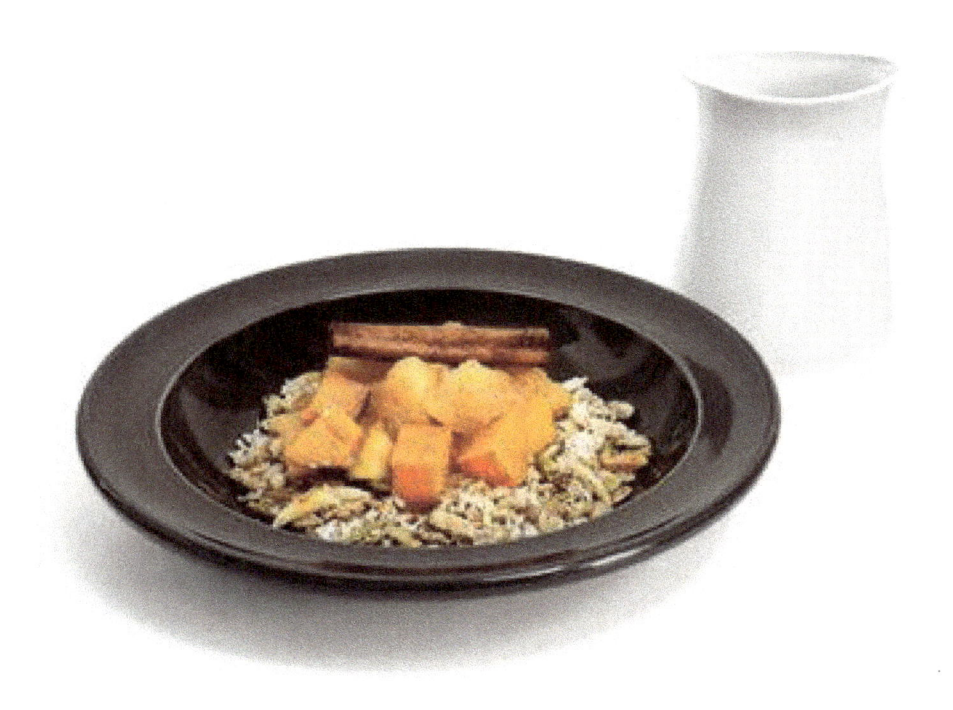

Braised Apples and Sweet Potato in Spiced Honey

1 Tbsp each, extra-virgin olive oil and unsalted butter

2 Granny Smith apples, cored, cut in ½-inch cubes, about 2 cups

1 medium yam, peeled and cut in ½-inch cubes, about 2 cups

1/3 cup honey

2 cinnamon sticks

½ tsp allspice

½ star anise

4 cups apple cider or apple juice

2 cups grain-free granola

1. In a large sauté pan, heat oil and butter over medium heat. Sauté the apple and yam cubes about 5 minutes or until slightly golden brown.

2. Meanwhile, in a medium saucepan on medium-low heat, add honey and let it slightly caramelize (turns copper color). Slowly stir in apple cider or juice, add spices, and reduce by one-third.

3. Lower heat to medium-low. Pour mixture over the apples and yams, and continue to cook until yams and apple cubes are tender but not falling apart. Remove cinnamon sticks and star anise before serving.

Grainless Granola

½ cup coconut oil

¼ tsp vanilla extract

1 tsp honey

¼ cup pumpkin seeds

¼ cup raw sesame seeds

¼ cup almond slivers

½ cup shredded coconut

1. In a small saucepan, melt coconut oil. Pour into large bowl. Add vanilla and honey, and stir. In a large frying pan on medium heat, roast pumpkin seeds until they pop, 2-3 minutes.

2. Remove from pan and set aside on paper towel. In the same pan, roast sesame seeds, almond slivers, and coconut until slightly brown, 2-3 minutes. Add pumpkin seeds and nut mixture to liquids and mix.

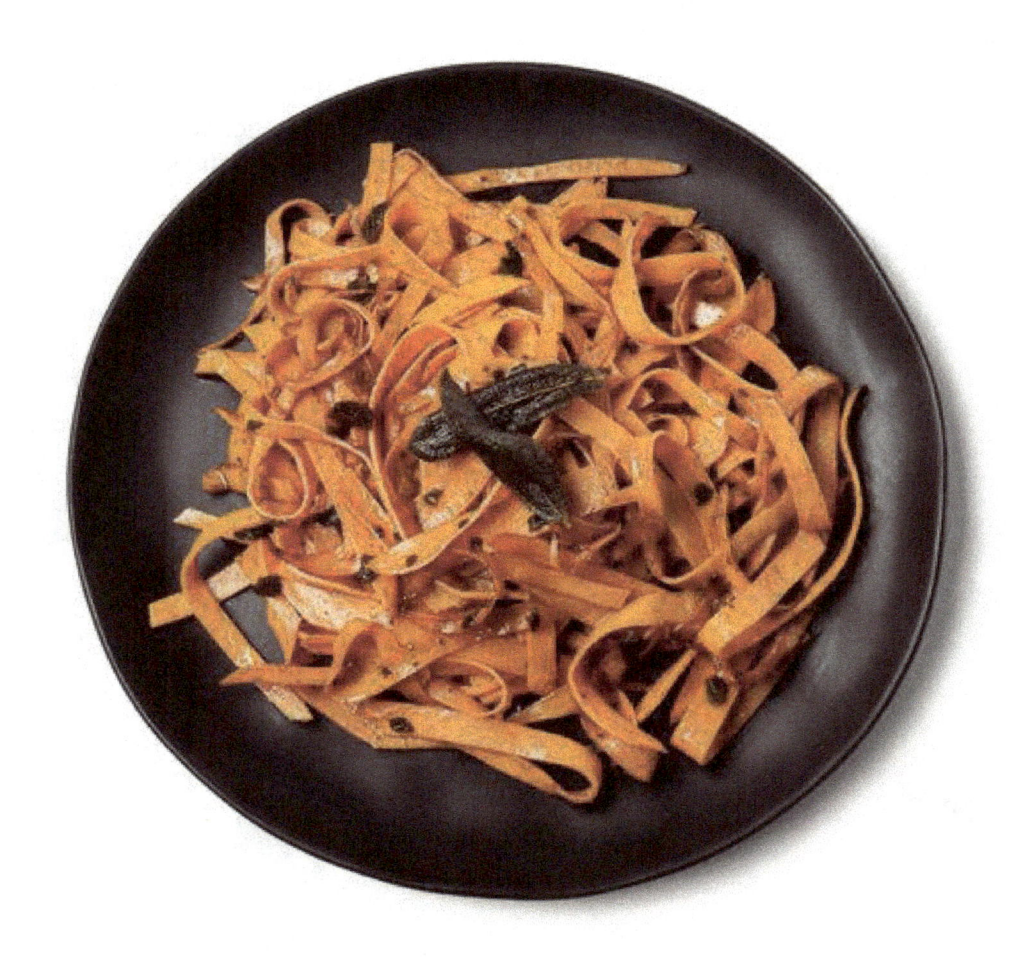

Sweet Potato Linguine with Sage and Brown Butter Sauce

Twirling a big, forkful of pasta is always so satisfying. Going paleo does not have to eliminate this pleasure. Sweet Potato Linguine rises above and beyond its pasta inspiration and takes less time than boiling a big pot of water.

Serves 2

    1 medium yam, long in shape

    1 Tbsp unsalted butter

    6 sage leaves (or more to taste)

    Kosher salt and freshly ground pepper to taste

1. Wash yam under running water and peel. Slice yam, lengthwise, as thinly as possible using a mandoline (a potato peeler does not slice thin enough).

2. Cut the long, thin slices into even strips about ¼-inch wide as linguine. Set aside.

3. In a large sauté pan, melt butter on medium-low heat and add the sage. Watch the butter closely as sage begins to brown (you don't want it to burn). When the sage is crisp, remove and set aside. Add the linguine-like strips to the butter and heat thoroughly. Stir and toss about 2–3 minutes. When tender and warmed through, plate and garnish with the fried sage.

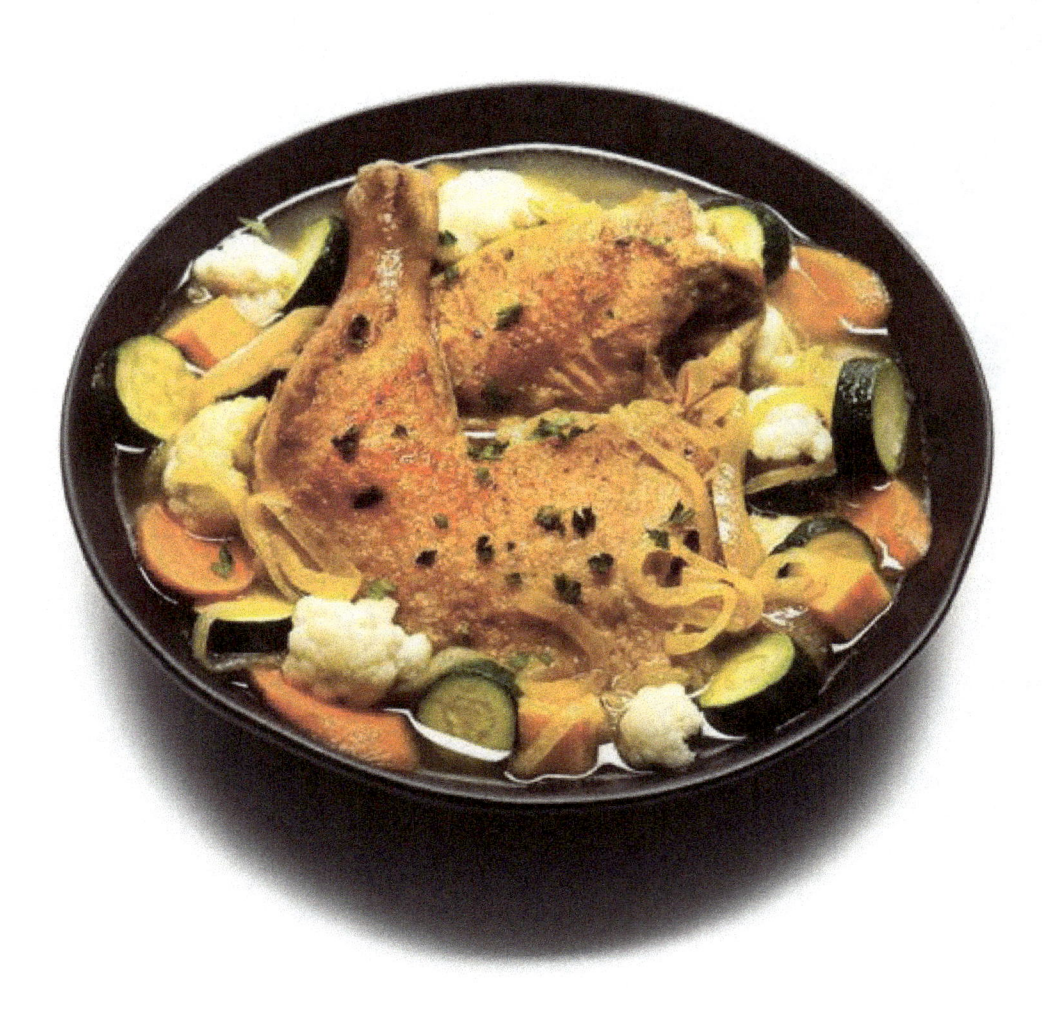

Moroccan Spiced Chicken

With Moroccan spices, chicken rises above the ordinary. Although pricey, saffron is a unique flavor that infuses food with a taste sure to delight. If there are any leftovers, the broth makes delicious soup. Cut the chicken off the bone and cut into bite-size pieces, add more vegetables, and cook until tender. Presto, another meal.

Serves 6

- 1 Tbsp each unsalted butter and extra-virgin olive oil
- 2 medium onions, thinly sliced
- ½ tsp ground ginger
- ½ tsp freshly ground black pepper
- 1 chicken, cut into 8-10 pieces
- 4–6 cups chicken broth, preferably homemade
- 1/8–1/4 tsp saffron
- 1–2 cinnamon sticks
- 1 tsp Kosher salt
- 2 carrots, peeled and cut into ½-inch slices
- 1 small yam, pealed and cut in ½-inch cubes, about 1 cup
- ½ head of cauliflower, cut into flowerets
- 2 zucchini, cut into ½-inch slices
- 3 Tbsp flat-leaf parsley, chopped

....

1. In a large frying pan, heat oil and butter over medium heat. Sauté the onion until softened. Add ginger and ground pepper. Stir to meld flavors. Remove onions to plate and set aside.

2. Add chicken pieces to the pan and cook until slightly browned. Add more oil if necessary. Add onion, chicken broth, saffron, cinnamon sticks, and salt. Bring to a slow boil, reduce heat, and simmer gently, covered for about 30 minutes or until chicken is almost done.

3. Add the carrots and simmer for 5 minutes. Add yam, cauliflower, and zucchini, and ½ of the parsley. Simmer for another 5 minutes or until vegetables are tender but don't fall apart. Garnish with remaining parsley and serve.

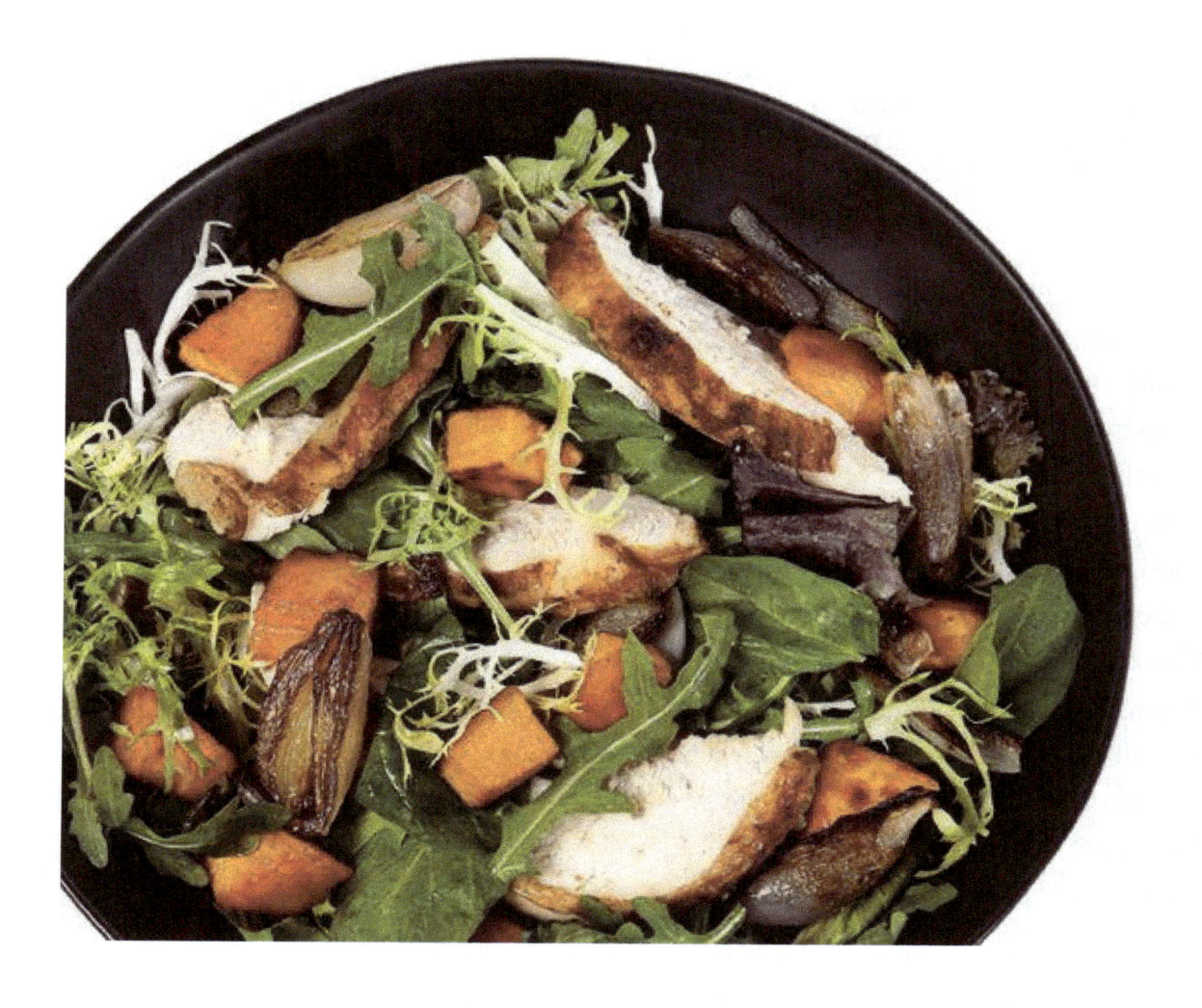

Salad with Roasted Chicken, Sweet Potato, and Shallots

This main course salad is filling and scrumptious. Brimming with grilled shallots, sweet potatoes, and roasted chicken, the salad will fill you up and satisfy with its deep flavors. To cut down on prep time and make salad assembly a snap, purchase a roasted chicken from the deli.

Serves 4

> 1 whole skinless, bone-in chicken breast, about 14 ounces or roasted chicken from deli
>
> 1/2 tsp ground ginger
>
> Kosher salt
>
> 4 Tbsp extra-virgin olive oil
>
> 2 Tbsp unsalted butter
>
> 2 medium yams, peeled and cut into ½-inch cubes, about 2 cups

8 shallots (same size), peeled and halved lengthwise or quartered if large

Mixed greens

2 Tbsp apple cider or apple vinegar

1 Tbsp fresh thyme leaves

Kosher salt and freshly ground pepper to taste

....

1. Preheat oven to 400 degrees. Rinse chicken and pat dry. Rub breast side with ginger and salt. In a large ovenproof skillet over medium heat, add 2 tablespoons of the oil and butter. Place chicken in skillet, breast side down; cook until breast side begins to turn golden brown, about 3-4 minutes.

2. Turn chicken over. Add yam and shallots to skillet; turn to coat in oil/butter. Transfer skillet to oven. Roast chicken and vegetables, turning vegetables at least once, until vegetables are tender and chicken is cooked through, 20–25 minutes. While chicken roasts, wash, spin dry, and put salad greens in serving bowl; set aside.

3. Transfer chicken to a cutting board and vegetables to a plate. Add apple vinegar or cider to skillet; cook over medium-high heat, scraping up brown bits from bottom of skillet with a wooden spoon. Remove from heat. Whisk in remaining olive oil and thyme. Salt and pepper to taste.

4. Cut chicken into ½-inch slices. Add chicken and vegetables to greens. Toss with warm vinaigrette and serve.

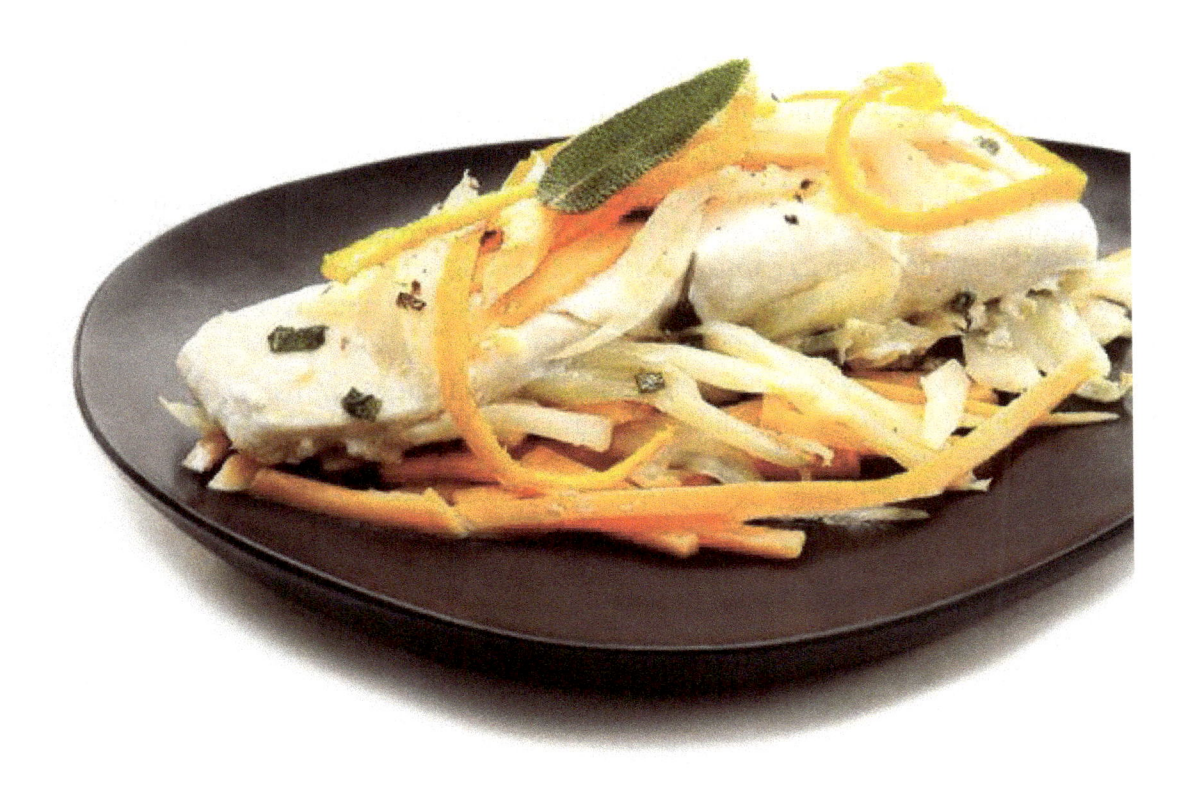

Halibut with Sweet Potato and Citrus

Baking in a tin foil packet can be a great tool to infuse flavors into delicate fish. Steamed in citrus, this halibut soaks up the essence of citrus mingled with sweet potato. The juice is packed with flavor. Spoon this goodness over the top before serving.

Serves 2

- 2 halibut filets
- 1 small yam, peeled
- 1 tsp extra-virgin olive oil
- ½ fresh fennel bulb
- 2 tsp fresh tarragon, chopped, plus whole leaves for garnish
- Zest of ½ orange, then squeezed for juice
- 1 tsp fresh ginger, grated
- Kosher salt and freshly ground pepper to taste

....

1. Heat oven to 350 degrees. Skin and debone halibut. Slice the yams and fennel lengthwise on a mandoline. Steam yam slices for 1 minute in a steamer with ½ cup water and remove. (Don't oversteam, the slices need to hold their shape.) In small sauté pan, heat oil to medium and sauté fennel with freshly cut tarragon for several minutes (until partly cooked but still crisp). Cut the fennel and yam into long ¼-inch strips.

2. Cut 2 pieces of aluminum foil into 12-inch squares. Place steamed slices of yam on aluminum foil. Add mixture of fennel and tarragon. Place halibut on top. Top halibut with strips of fennel and yam as garnish. Add small amount of chopped tarragon and orange zest. Add teaspoon of oil to the orange juice, whisk, and pour over top. Sprinkle grated ginger over top. Salt and pepper to taste.

3. Loosely fold the foil over the halibut. Bake for 10-15 minutes until fish is opaque. Plate, spoon liquid over fish, and garnish with tarragon.

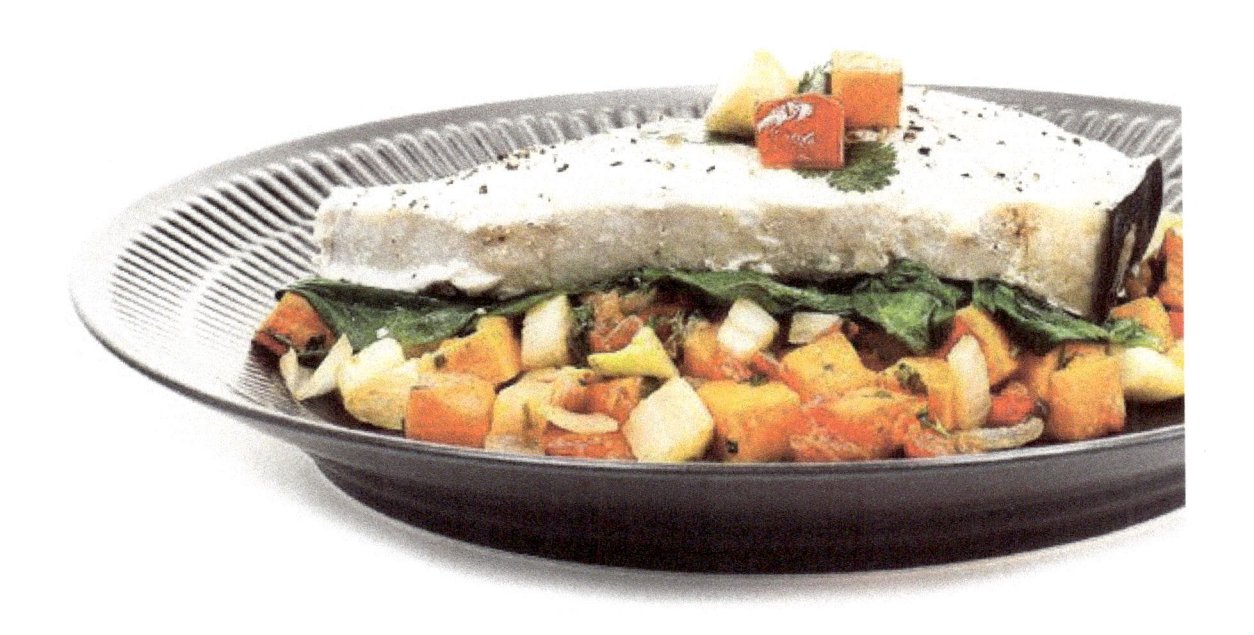

Swordfish with Sweet Potato Salsa

High on flavor and texture, this salsa is a fine accompaniment to dress up white fish. Baking the fish in tin foil packets makes cooking a cinch.

Serves 4

- 2 Tbsp extra-virgin olive oil
- 1 small onion, diced, about ½ cup
- 1 small yam, peeled and cut in ½-inch cubes, about 1 cup
- ½ fennel, core removed, diced, about ½ cup
- ½ a red bell pepper, core and seeds removed, diced, about ½ cup
- 2 medium cloves garlic, crushed
- Pinch of chili flakes
- 6 slices prosciutto or bacon, chopped (kitchen scissors make it easier), fried until crisp
- 1 small tomato, seeds removed, diced, about ½ cup
- ½ cup cilantro, chopped
- 6-oz bag of baby spinach leaves
- ½ lemon
- Kosher salt and freshly ground pepper to taste
- 4 firm, white fish filets such as swordfish, halibut, sea bass, skinned and deboned

1. Preheat oven to 350 degrees. In a large frying pan, heat oil on medium. Add onion, yam, fennel, and red bell pepper. Season with salt and pepper, add crushed garlic. Sauté lightly for 1–2 minutes (don't overcook, salsa should remain crunchy).

2. Meanwhile, in a small frying pan, crisp the prosciutto or bacon. To the onion mixture, add tomato, ½ of the cilantro, ½ of the prosciutto or bacon, and chili flakes. Stir to blend flavors. Adjust seasoning.

3. Cut two pieces of aluminum foil into 12-inch squares. Place a handful of spinach on each piece of foil. Sprinkle with oil, lemon juice, salt, and pepper. Place the filet on top. Sprinkle with oil and lemon juice. Top with a generous spoonful of salsa. Garnish with remaining prosciutto and cilantro. Loosely close aluminum packet and bake for 10-15 minutes or until fish is done.

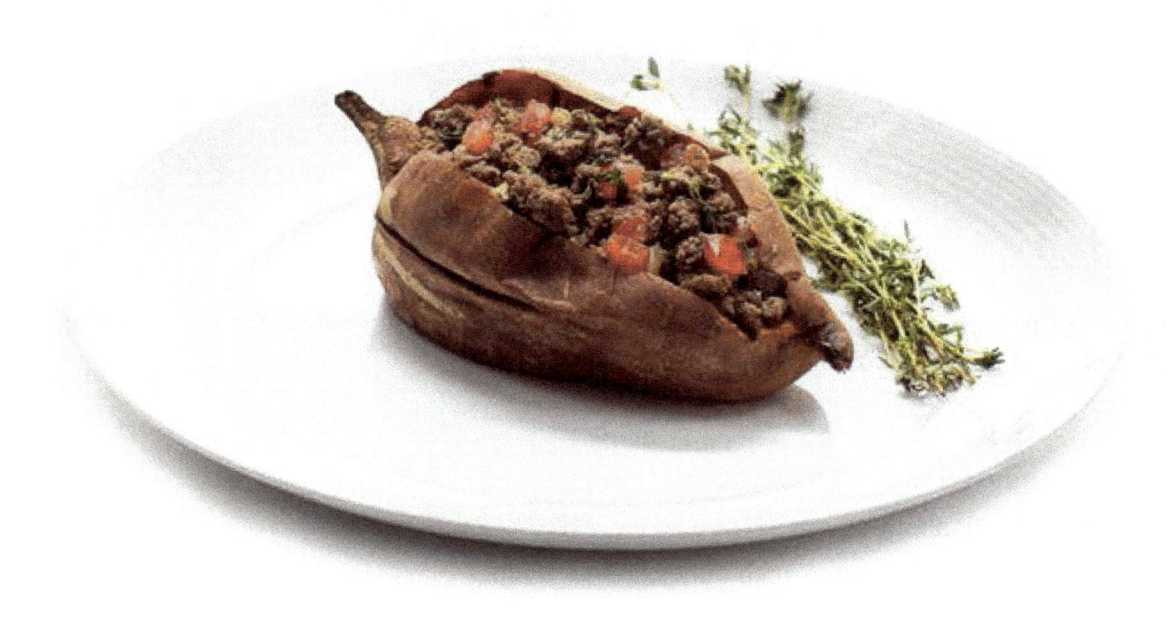

Stuffed Sweet Potato Three Ways

The time has come to elevate this humble root to the main attraction of the dinner plate. Topping the smart carb sweet potato with good protein is an easy way to create a well-rounded meal. Here are three versions that play with different meat stuffing and spices so you don't get bored. The baked sweet potatoes and stuffing can be made ahead so all that is needed at the last minute is to stuff and reheat.

Baked Yam

Serves 2-3

2-3 medium yams

1. Select medium yams of about the same size. Scrub under running water and place on a baking sheet covered with aluminum foil in a 400-degree oven. Bake until soft (easily pierced with a fork), about 1 hour. Create a pocket in the middle and fill with chosen meat mixture. If needed place in a baking dish, cover with aluminum foil, and put in a 350-degree oven for an additional 15 minutes or until heated through.

....

Beef Sausage Filling for Baked Yam

1 Tbsp extra-virgin olive oil

½ medium onion, diced

2 garlic cloves, diced

½ lb ground beef

¼ lb ground pork sausage

1 medium tomato, seeded and chopped

2–3 tsp fresh thyme

4 Tbsp fresh cilantro, chopped fine, reserve 1 Tbsp for finish

½ tsp herbs de Provence

½ tsp cumin

Kosher salt and freshly ground pepper to taste

1. In a large frying pan, heat oil and butter over medium. Sauté onion 1 minute. Add garlic and sauté lightly. Set aside on a plate. In the same pan, sauté beef and sausage until partly brown. Set aside on separate plate.

2. Return onion and garlic to the pan. Add tomato, thyme, and 3 tablespoons of the cilantro. Mix well and cook 1-2 minutes. Add beef mixture and remaining seasonings to the pan, continue cooking another 5 minutes. Adjust seasoning to taste. If necessary add a small amount of water to keep the mixture moist. Stir in remaining cilantro and stuff yams.

Pork Sausage Filling for Baked Yam

1 Tbsp extra-virgin olive oil

½ medium onion, diced

½ a fennel bulb, with core removed, diced

2 garlic cloves, diced

¼ red bell pepper, diced, about 4 Tbsp

2–3 tsp fresh thyme or ½ tsp dried

Kosher salt and freshly ground pepper

¾ lb ground pork sausage

....

1. In a large frying pan, heat oil on medium and sauté onion and fennel, approximately 1 minute. Add garlic, red pepper, and ½ of the herbs. Sauté several minutes to blend flavors. Salt and pepper to taste. Remove to plate.

2. In the same pan, add sausage and brown until cooked, stirring frequently. Remove excess fat. Return onion mixture to the pan and continue to cook about 5 minutes. Add remaining fresh thyme. Add small amount of water if necessary to keep the mixture moist. Adjust seasoning to taste and stuff yams. If needed, cover with aluminum foil and place in 350 degree oven to heat through.

Lamb Sausage Filling for Baked Yam

1 Tbsp extra-virgin olive oil

½ medium onion, diced

2 garlic cloves, diced

½ lb ground lamb

¼ lb ground pork sausage

1 small eggplant, cut into small cubes, about 2 cups

4–5 brown or white mushrooms, sliced

1½–2 tsp fresh rosemary, finely chopped or ½ tsp dried

5–6 dried apricots, diced

Kosher salt and freshly ground pepper to taste

....

1. In large frying pan, heat oil on medium heat and sauté onion approximately 1 minute. Reduce heat and add garlic, sauté lightly. Set aside on plate. Increase heat to medium, sauté the lamb and sausage, until partly brown, and then set aside on separate plate. Remove any excess fat from the pan.

2. Add small amount of oil and return onion to the pan. Add eggplant, mushrooms, and half the rosemary. Mix well and cook several minutes.

3. Return meat to the pan with onion mixture, add dried apricots, remaining rosemary, and seasonings. Cook for several minutes. Turn heat to medium-low, add a small amount of water if necessary and cook to blend flavors, about 5 minutes. Salt and pepper to taste. Stuff yams. If needed cover with aluminum foil and place in 350 degree oven to heat through.

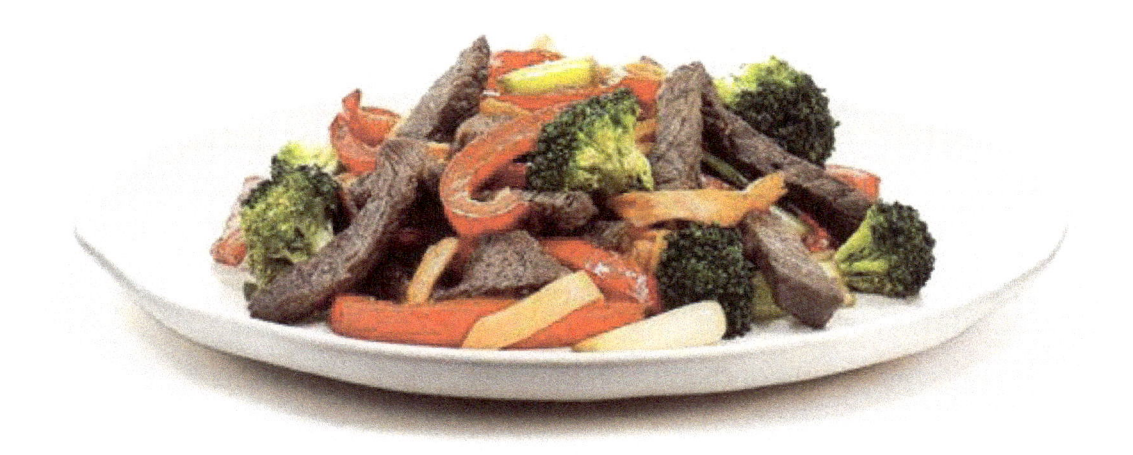

Spicy Beef with Pepper and Sweet Potato

Easy and reliably delicious, stir-fry recipes are a great way to get dinner on the table in a flash. While some stir-fry ingredients may be high in soy, fructose, and other mystery ingredients, this stir-fry has all the flavor without the hidden sugars. Serve over cauliflower rice.

Serves 4

    1 piece of flank steak (1 lb)

    1 Tbsp gluten-free soy sauce

    1 Tbsp Chinese rice vinegar

    1 Tbsp sesame oil

    1 Tbsp garlic, peeled and finely grated (use a rasp grater)

    1 Tbsp fresh ginger, finely grated (use a rasp grater)

    ½ tsp Kosher salt

    4 Tbsp coconut oil

    1 small yam, peeled and thinly sliced lengthwise on a mandoline, about 1 cup

    1 large red bell pepper, cut into thin strips, about 1 cup

    3 scallions, halved lengthwise and cut into 1-inch pieces

    1 cup broccoli florets

    2–3 tsp chili garlic sauce

1 head of cauliflower

1. Cut steak into 1/4-inch strips. In a medium bowl, add soy sauce, rice vinegar, sesame oil, garlic, ginger, salt, and stir. Add steak strips and marinate 20–30 minutes. Cut, sliced yams into thin strips about 1/4-inch wide.

2. In large frying pan or wok, heat 2 tablespoons oil over high heat. Add beef, spreading in one layer. Cook beef undisturbed to brown, 1 minute, then stir-fry until meat is just brown but still pink in center, about 1 minute. Transfer meat and any juices to plate.

3. Pour remaining 2 tablespoons oil in pan and heat on high. Add yam, bell pepper, scallions, and broccoli. Salt to taste. Stir-fry 1 minute, add re-served beef with any juices and chili garlic sauce. Stir-fry until combined well. Transfer to platter and serve if desired over Cauliflower Rice.

4. Cauliflower Rice: cut one head of cauliflower into small florets. Steam briefly, 2–3 minutes. Run the florets through the food processor, using the grating blade. Add Kosher salt and unsalted butter to taste.

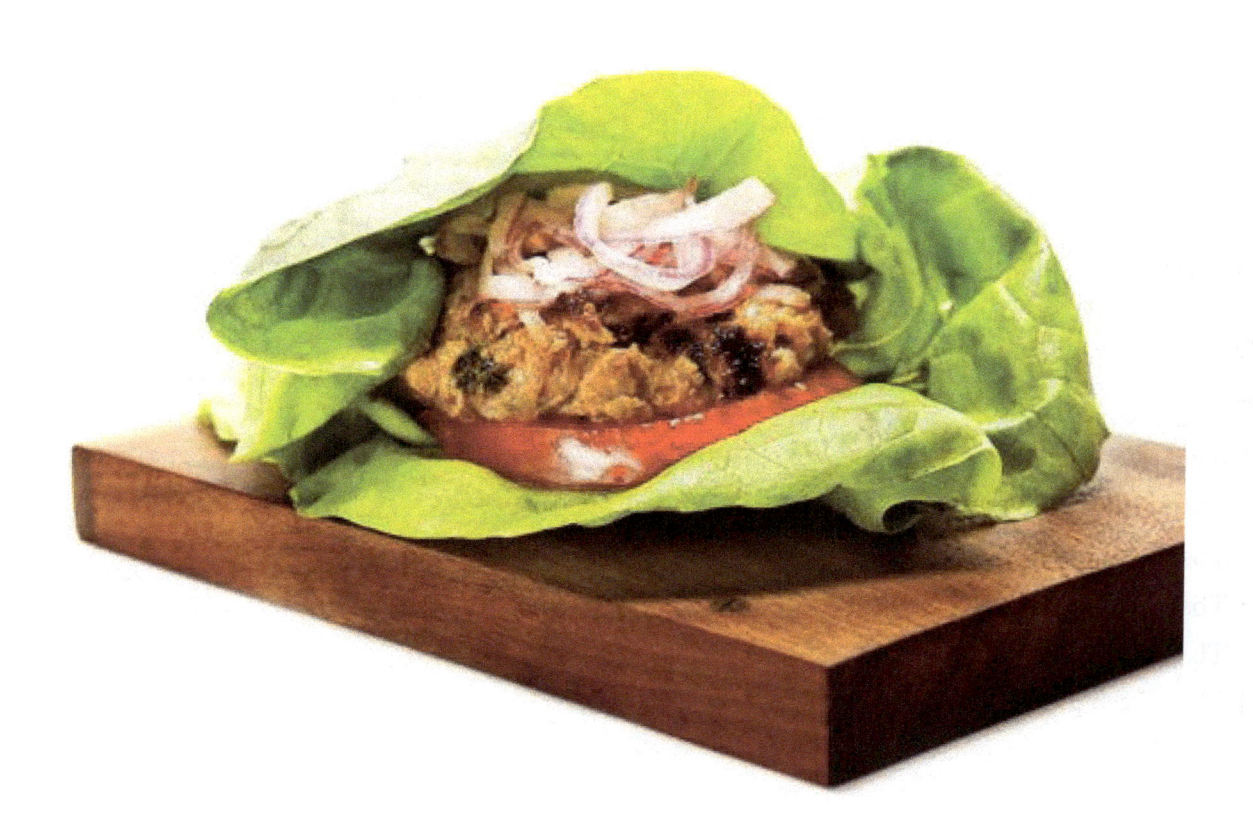

Turkey Burger Cookies

How do you improve a simple meat patty? Turkey cookies are a caramelized, gooey burger that is more like a cookie than a main course. To retain caramelized goodness, these are better done in a pan than on the grill. Due the natural sugars in the sweet potatoes, these patties tend to brown/burn faster than meat counterparts. Keep a close eye on them until you get the timing down.

Serves 2

- 1 lb ground turkey
- ½ onion, finely chopped
- 1 cup yam or Japanese Satsumaimo mash
- 1 tsp fresh thyme, chopped
- ¼-½ tsp ground cumin, depending on taste
- Kosher salt and freshly ground pepper
- 1 tsp unsalted butter
- Tomatoes and red onion, sliced
- Butter lettuce

....

1. To make mash: Heat oven to 400 degrees. Place medium yam or Satsumaimo on baking sheet and bake for 1 hour or until easily pierced with a fork. Cool, scoop out flesh from skin. Discard skin. Purée flesh in food processor. (Mash can be made days ahead and frozen or refrigerated until ready to use.)

2. In a large mixing bowl, add turkey, onions, mash, spices, salt, and pepper. Mix gently. Form mixture into patties.

3. In a large frying pan, heat butter to medium-low. Place patties in pan and cook for 5 minutes. Flip and cover pan. Watch carefully so they don't burn.

4. Continue cooking until done. Place tomato and onion on top of patty. Wrap in large pieces of lettuce and serve with your favorite aoli or condiments.

Hearty Vegetable Soup

The broth is the heart of any soup. Master chefs know that the extra step of simmering stock with leeks, carrots, and onions infuses the base with deep, rich flavor. If you don't have the time to do this step, skip the recipe until you do. The extra effort makes the difference between a soup that is out of this world and just so-so.

Serves 4

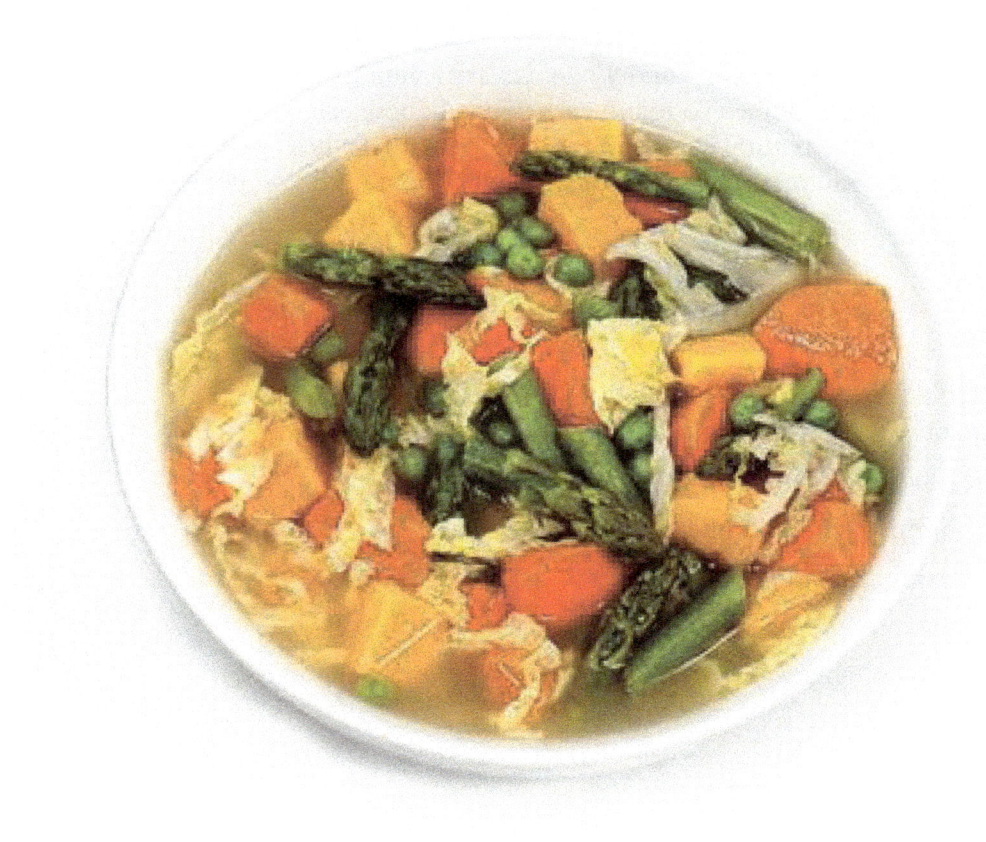

3 Tbsp extra-virgin olive oil

2 cups carrots, peeled and thinly sliced

2 cups leeks, quartered, cleaned, coarsely chopped, white and light green

2 cups onions, coarsely chopped

Kosher salt and freshly ground black pepper

8 cups chicken stock, preferably homemade

1 bay leaf

3 sprigs thyme

1 clove garlic, crushed

10 peppercorns, crushed

1 medium yam, peeled and cut into ½-inch cubes, about 2 cups

1 cup carrots, peeled and sliced, ½-inch thick

8 oz asparagus, tough ends removed, cut into 1-inch pieces on diagonal

1 cup green beans, ends removed and cut into 1-inch pieces on diagonal

1 cup peas

1 small head Savoy cabbage, quartered and sliced

Extra-virgin olive oil for drizzle

Flat-leaf parsley leaves

....

1. For the broth: Heat oil in an 8- to 10-quart pot over medium. Add carrots, leeks, and onions, and stir to coat in the oil. Season with salt and pepper. Reduce heat to medium-low and cook 30–35 minutes until vegetables are slightly cooked. Add the chicken stock, bay leaf, thyme, peppercorns, and garlic. Increase heat and bring to a simmer. Simmer for 20 minutes. Strain the broth into another pot. Discard the vegetables and herbs. Set broth aside.

2. For the soup: Place yams, carrots, and a pinch of salt in a medium pot, cover with cold water, and bring to a simmer. Cook for 4 to 5 minutes, or until vegetables are tender but slightly resistant. Drain.

3. Bring a large pot of salted water to a boil. Have ready a bowl of water ice. Put asparagus into strainer, immerse in boiling water and blanch for 1 minute. Remove and pour asparagus into the ice bath. Repeat with the green beans, 3 minutes; the peas, 1 minute. Add cabbage to the boiling water and blanch just until tender. Chill in ice bath. Drain all the blanched vegetables.

4. Bring the broth to a simmer. Adjust seasoning. Add the blanched vegetables and return to simmer to heat vegetables. Remove from heat and serve, drizzled with olive oil and garnished with parsley leaves.

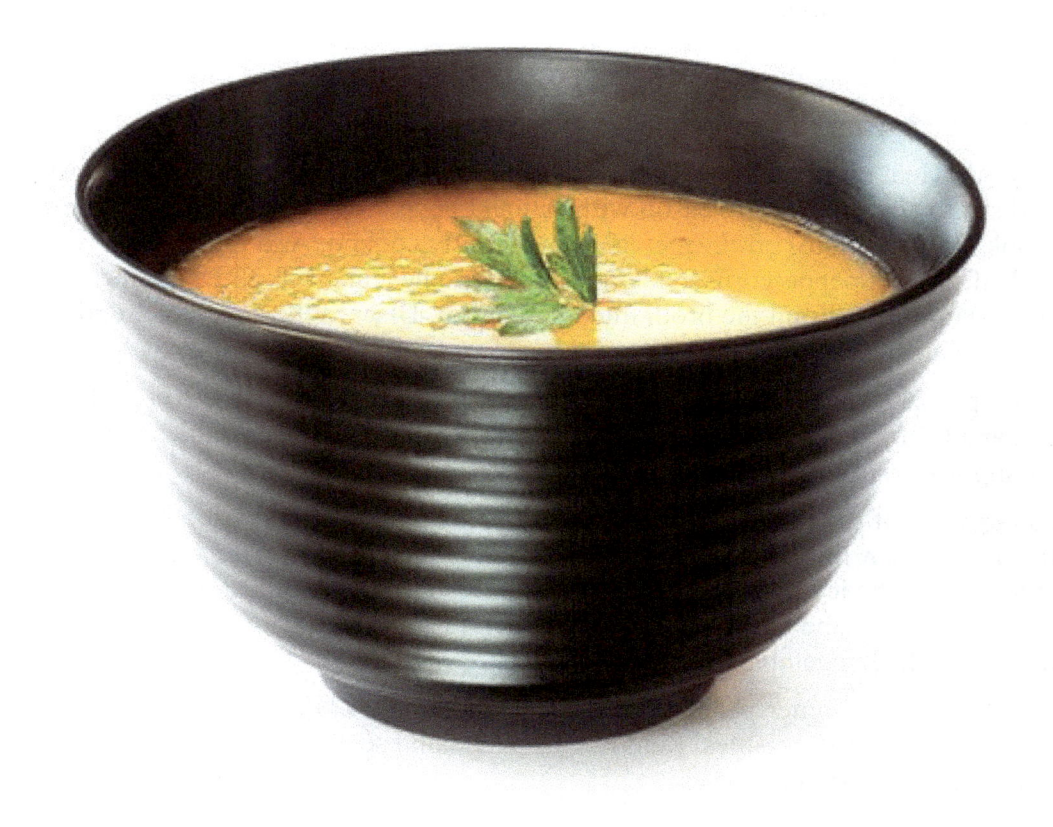

Sopa de Batata Doce

Cream soups are a staple of crisp, fall nights. This simple soup from Brazil packs all the comfort of a warm bowl without the cream. Quality tomatoes, such as heirlooms, intensify the flavor.

Serves 6

- 1 lb white sweet potatoes
- 4 Tbsp unsalted butter
- 1 medium onion, finely chopped
- 4 medium flavorful tomatoes, such as heirloom, peeled, seeded, and chopped
- 4 cups beef stock
- Kosher salt and freshly ground pepper to taste
- 2 tsp chopped parsley

1. Peel the sweet potatoes, thickly slice, put into a 2 quart saucepan, and cover with cold, salted water. Bring to a boil, reduce heat, and simmer covered until tender, about 20 minutes. Drain and chop coarsely.

2. In a large frying pan, heat butter on medium. Sauté the onion until translucent. Add the tomatoes and cook for about 5 minutes longer. Put the mixture into a blender or food processor with the sweet potatoes and 1 cup of the stock. Reduce to a smooth purée.

3. Pour purée and rest of stock into saucepan. Season with salt and pepper and reheat. Garnish with chopped parsley.

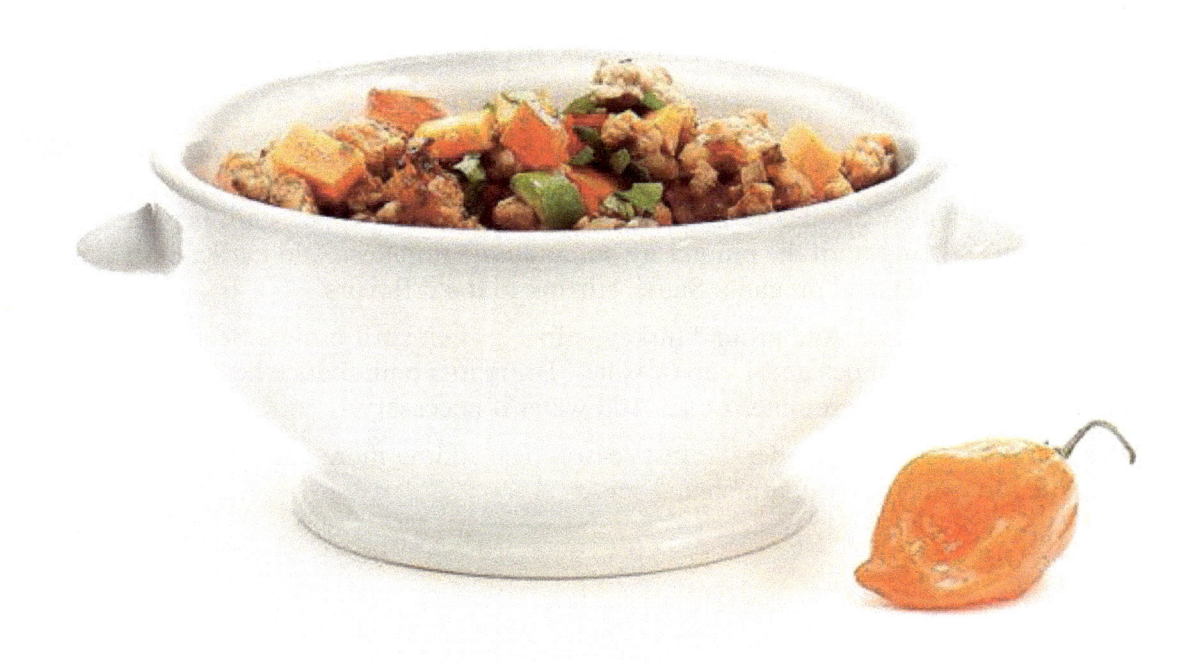

Southwestern Chili

Every cook needs a chili soup standby. Chili without beans, however, can seem incomplete and leaves something to be desired. Using yams provides the heartiness with good carbs. Monterey Jack cheese, sour cream, and chopped fresh cilantro make good garnishes.

Serves 6

> 2 Tbsp palm oil
>
> 1 yellow onion, diced
>
> 1 green pepper, veins and seeds removed, diced

2–3 fresh jalapeño peppers, seeded and minced (serranos if more heat desired)

1 celery stalk, sliced ¼-inch thick

4 cloves of garlic, minced

1 Tbsp chili powder

2½ tsp ground cumin

¼ tsp cayenne pepper

¾ tsp dried oregano

1 lb ground chicken or turkey

Kosher salt and freshly ground black pepper

2 (28-ounce) cans diced plum (Roma) tomatoes

1 small yam, peeled and cut into ½-inch cubes, about 1 cup

Garnishes—Monterrey jack cheese, sour cream, and cilantro

••

1. In a large frying pan, heat oil over medium. Add onion, green pepper, chili peppers, and celery. Sauté, stirring until the onions are soft, about 5 minutes. Add garlic, chili powder, cumin, cayenne, and oregano. Sauté, stirring to meld flavors.

2. Increase heat to medium. Add ground turkey, stirring often until brown. Season with salt and pepper. Add tomatoes and 1 cup of water. Bring to a boil, reduce heat to low, cover, and simmer for thirty minutes or so. Add water if necessary.

3. Add yam and simmer until tender. Adjust seasonings, adding more chili powder if desired. Ladle into soup bowls, garnish and serve.

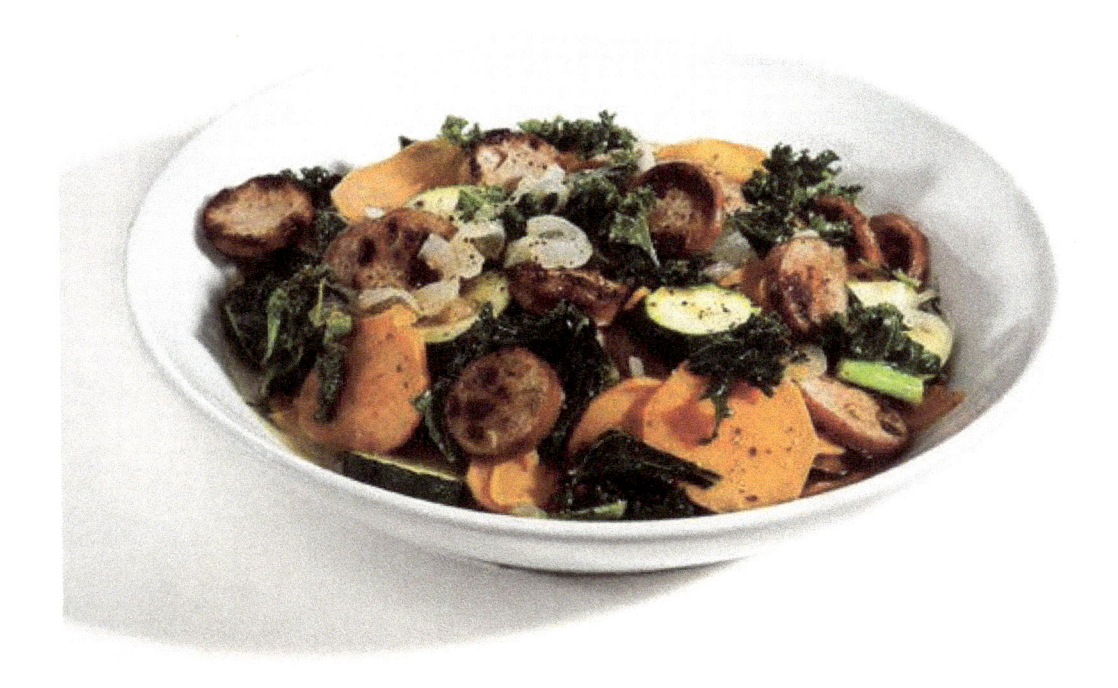

One-Pan Scramble with Sweet Potato

When dinner needs to be made and served fast, nutrition and taste need not be sacrificed. This one-pan meal is easy to prepare and cooks in a flash. Add other veggies lingering in your fridge—the more the merrier.

Serves 4

    4 Aidells Chicken Apple Sausages or favorite sausage, sliced into ½-inch pieces

    1 cup chicken or vegetable broth, preferably homemade or organic, low sodium

    ½ onion, thinly sliced

    2 cloves garlic, chopped

    Handful of kale or chard, chopped, tough stems removed

    1 zucchini, sliced into ½-inch pieces

    1 small yam, peeled and thinly sliced crosswise, about 1 cup

Kosher salt and freshly ground pepper to taste

Hot pepper flakes (optional)

....

1. In a large sauté pan on medium heat, slightly brown sausage slices. Remove to plate.

2. In the same pan, heat broth over medium-high. Add onion, garlic, kale or chard, and season with salt and pepper. Cover with lid and simmer 5-10 minutes or until kale or chard is tender.

3. Add zucchini and sweet potato slices and simmer for a few minutes until slices are cooked through. Add sausage to the mixture and heat. Adjust seasoning. Add hot pepper flakes if desired and serve.

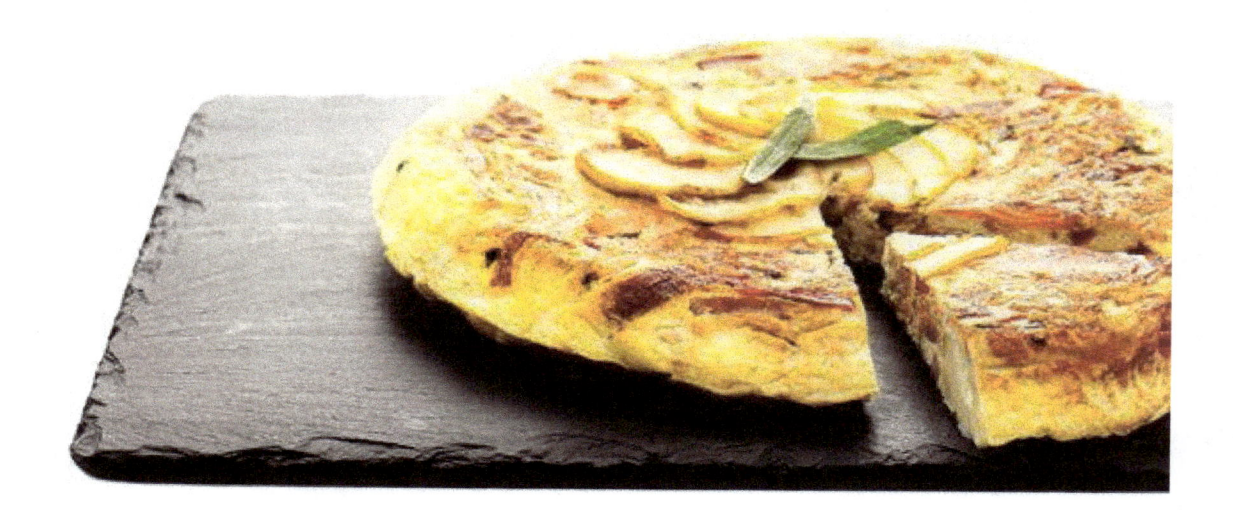

Sweet Potato Frittata

This frittata is packed with flavor and sure to chase egg boredom away. Serve hot or cold; it keeps well in the refrigerator to enjoy for days. A warning: it's so good, even with the best intentions, the Sweet Potato Frittata won't last long.

Serves 6

4 tsp extra-virgin olive oil

1 medium yam, peeled and cut crosswise into thin slices

½ large yellow onion, cut in thin slices

¼ sweet red bell pepper, cut in thin strips

1 tsp thyme or more to taste

½ small ham steak cut into thin pieces, ½-inch long, about ½ cup

½ of 3-ounce package of chopped pancetta

Kosher salt and freshly ground pepper

1 small jar quartered marinated artichoke hearts or bottoms

5 sprigs tarragon, 3 chopped and 2 reserved for garnish

6–8 springs parsley, chopped (need a good handful)

6 eggs

½ apple, Granny Smith or other tart variety

2–3 Tbsp unsalted butter

··

1. In a large sauté pan, heat 2 teaspoons of oil on medium-low. Add yam slices and sauté 1-2 minutes. Remove to plate.

2. In the same pan, heat 1 teaspoon oil on medium. Sauté onion and pepper for 3–4 minutes until onions are translucent. Sprinkle with thyme. Add yam to onion mixture. Salt and pepper. Continue to cook.

3. Meanwhile, place chopped ham and pancetta in a small sauté pan with 1 teaspoon oil and cook over medium heat for 5 minutes until slightly brown. Add to yam mixture. Add more oil if needed. Season with salt and pepper to taste. Cook until the yam slices are mostly cooked through but are still firm enough to retain their shape. Add the artichokes, chopped tarragon, and parsley. Turn the mixture carefully.

4. Beat eggs in a bowl. Add eggs to the yam mixture. Allow the eggs to seep to the bottom of the pan by opening up the yam mixture with spatula. Cook the frittata on medium heat, running the spatula along the pan rim to separate the tortilla from the pan. Repeat several times. After a few minutes, lower the heat to prevent burning and to ensure the eggs cook evenly.

5. Cook until the sides are firm and lightly browned (the top of the frittata should be mostly cooked, but only firm enough to turn and still runny in parts).

6. Slice ½ apple into thin slices. In a small sauté pan, melt a tablespoon of butter over medium-low heat. Add a sprig of tarragon for flavoring. Add the finely-sliced apples and cook over medium heat until apples are slightly brown.

7. When the frittata is cooked on one side and ready to turn, place a dinner plate or other flat lid over the pan and invert frying pan. Slide the frittata, uncooked side down back into the pan to finish cooking, approximately 3–5 minutes. Once the frittata has finished cooking, slide it onto a serving platter. Altogether the tortilla should take approximately 15–20 minutes after the eggs have been added.

8. Decorate the top of the tortilla with the apple slices using a circular pattern and add sprigs of tarragon before serving.

Rainbow Cubes

So simple, so delicious. Rainbow cubes are a great on-the-go treat to keep you going. Kids will love the color. All will love the taste. It's amazing such goodness can come straight from the ground. The purple variety can be found in Chinese/Japanese markets.

Serving: 2–3 cups

- 1 small Okinawa sweet potato (purple), peeled and cut into ½-inch cubes
- 1 small sweet potato (white), peeled and cut into ½-inch cubes
- 1 small yam, peeled and cut into ½-inch cubes
- Extra-virgin olive oil
- Kosher salt and freshly ground pepper to taste

....

1. Preheat oven to 425 degrees. Place cubes in large mixing bowl and drizzle with oil. Toss to ensure even coverage. Salt and pepper generously.

2. Spread cubes in one layer on baking sheet so they do not touch. Bake for approximately 30-35 minutes, flipping cubes half way through. Watch carefully to avoid burning. Once cubes are crispy on the outside and tender on the inside, remove from the oven and cool.

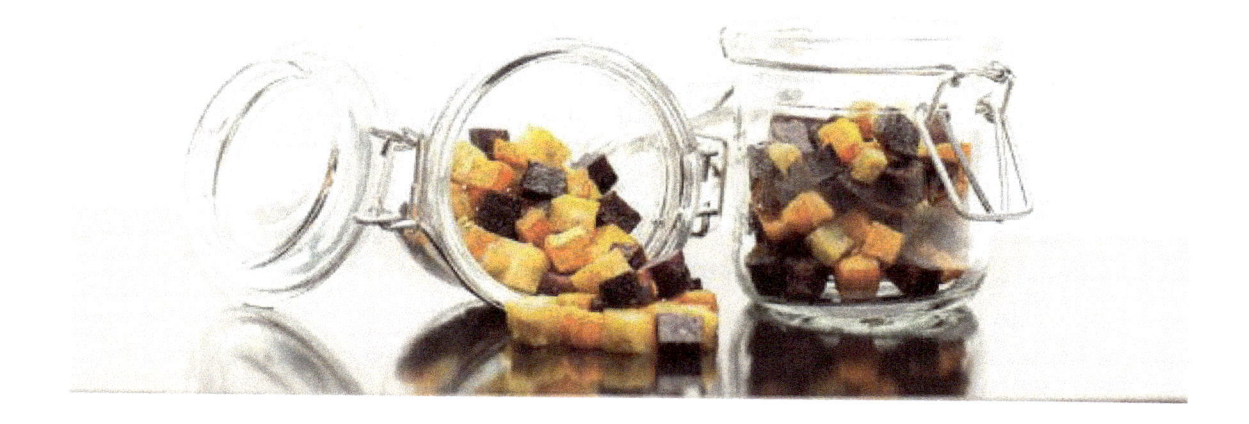

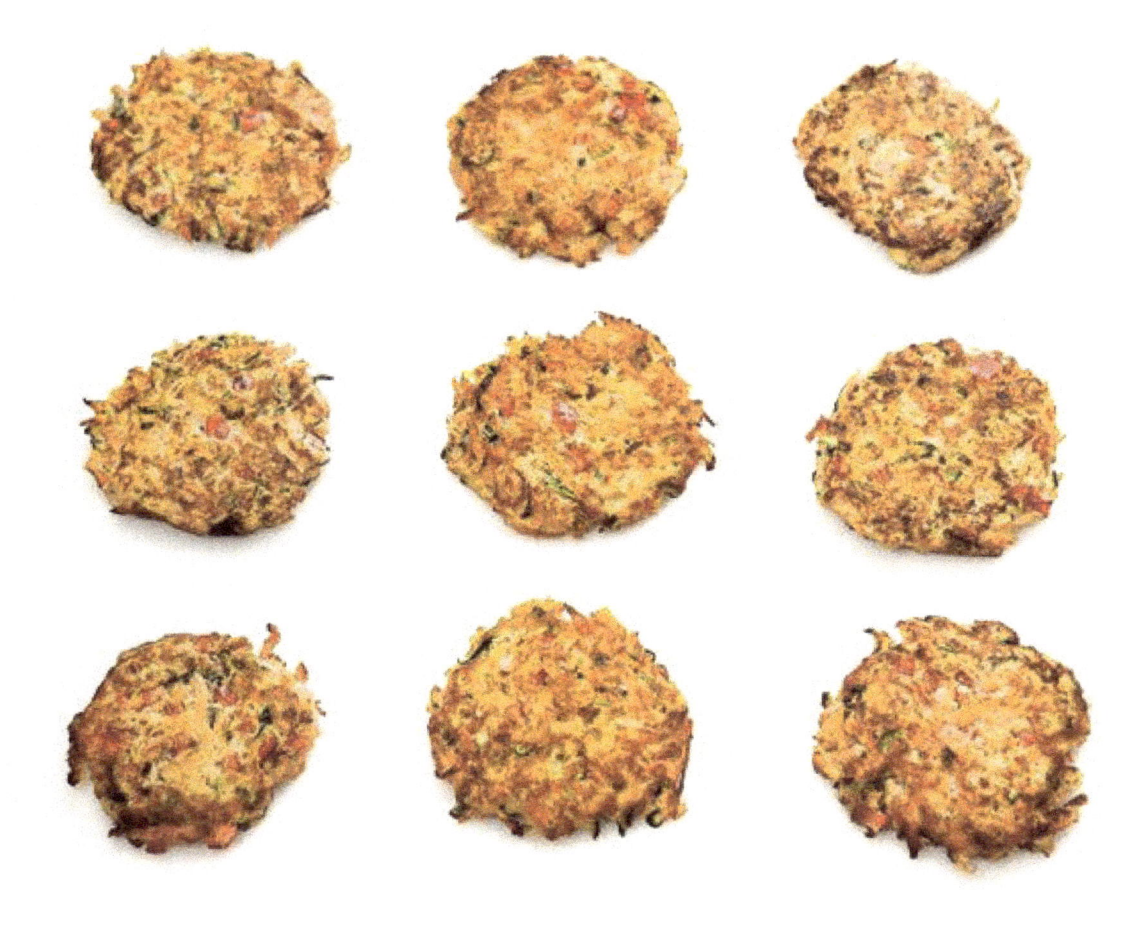

Sweet Potato Vegetable Latkes

Even the biggest vegetable critics will fall in love with these patties. Packed with a combination of nature's goodies, these latkes are sweet, satisfying, and quick to make.

Serves 6

- 1 large egg
- 3 Tbsp almond flour
- 1 tsp dried tarragon or fresh, chopped
- 2 tsp chives, chopped fine
- Kosher salt and freshly ground pepper to taste
- 2/3 cup yam, peeled and shredded

1/3 cup zucchini, shredded

¼ cup carrot, shredded

1 Tbsp onion, diced

2 cloves of garlic, diced fine

2 Tbsp red bell pepper, diced

1 Tbsp extra-virgin olive oil

....

1. In a large bowl, mix egg, almond flour, tarragon, chives, salt, and pepper. Add the yam, zucchini, carrot, onion, garlic, and bell pepper. Mix well. The batter will be runny.

2. In a large sauté pan, heat oil on medium-low. Drop generous tablespoons of the mixture or desired size latkes into the pan.

3. Flatten slightly into patty shape. Cover and cook until brown. Turn over, replace lid, and cook until lightly browned and vegetables are cooked (a couple of minutes per side).

Sweet Potato Poppers

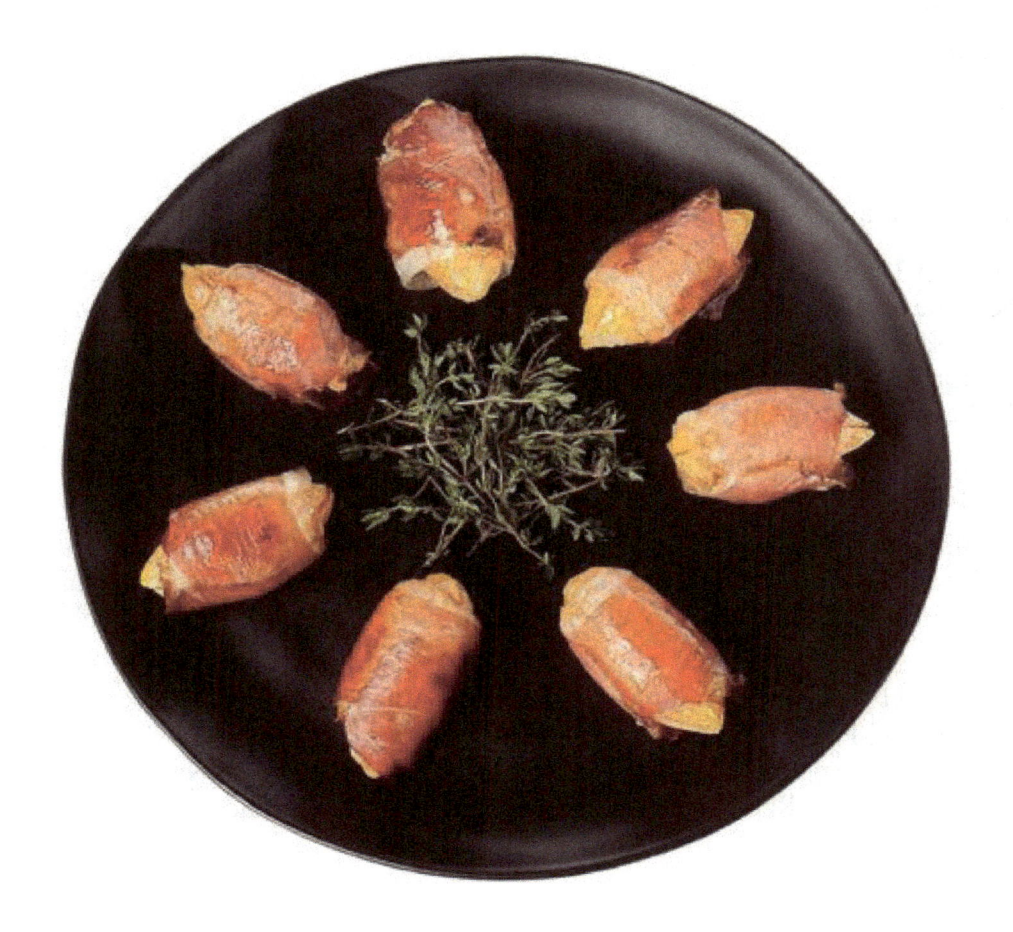

Sweet Potato Poppers are small in size and big on flavor. A combination of herby, savory, and sweet, they delight the taste buds. Poppers make an ideal appetizer—fun to pass around at a gathering of friends.

Serves 6

    6 very small yams, peeled to same size

    ¼ cup crumbled blue cheese or feta cheese

    ½ tsp fresh rosemary, minced

    1 tsp fresh thyme, minced

3 fresh sage leaves, minced

1 clove garlic, minced

Kosher salt and freshly ground black pepper to taste

3–4 oz prosciutto

1 Tbsp extra-virgin oil

....

1. Preheat oven to 375 degrees. Peel yams until they are sized for three or four bites each and the same size for even cooking. Save the peelings for another use. Place the yams in a large saucepan, cover with water. Salt water liberally and bring to boil. Parboil yams for 5 minutes or until knife pierces with slight resistance. Potatoes will not be cooked completely but will finish cooking in the oven. Drain and cool.

2. Meanwhile, in small bowl, combine cheese, herbs, garlic, salt, and pepper. Mash with a fork until fully incorporated. Taste and adjust seasonings. Set aside.

3. Halve the yams. Using a melon ball, scoop out a shallow trough 1-inch long down the middle of each half. Fill with 1 teaspoon of cheese-herb mixture. Place the top half over bottom. Gently place the halves together so the stuffing doesn't seep out when baked.

4. Wrap each stuffed yam tightly with thinly sliced prosciutto, working carefully so the prosciutto doesn't rip. Place the poppers on a sheet pan lined with aluminum foil and drizzle with oil. Cook poppers for 10 minutes, then turn 1/4. Cook for another 15 minutes, turning 1/4 again. Repeat until all sides are crisp, browned, and easily pierced with fork. Serve warm.

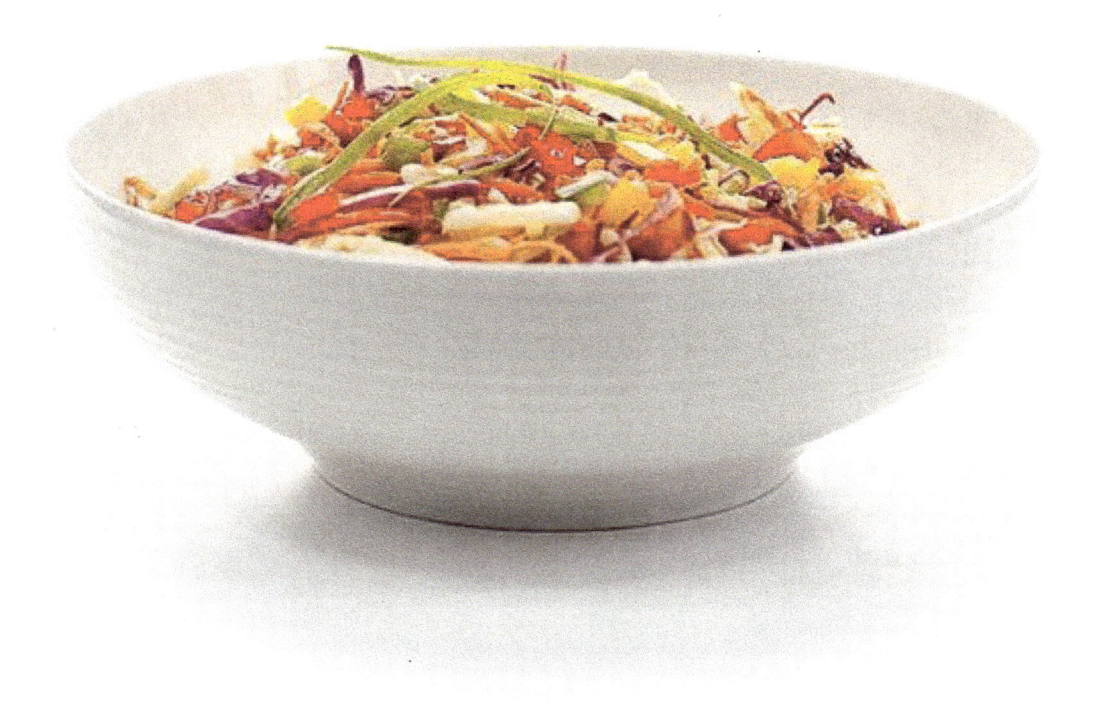

Sweet Potato Slaw

Make this colorful slaw ahead to let flavors meld and mix. Unlike green salads, a big batch keeps well in the fridge for days. A showpiece on the dinner table or great afternoon snack, Sweet Potato Slaw gets better with time.

Serves 8

   2 cups shredded cabbage, about ½ cabbage

   1 cup shredded red cabbage, about ¼ cabbage

   1 medium yellow bell pepper, cored, seeded, and thinly sliced

   1 medium red bell pepper, cored, seeded, and thinly sliced

   ½ medium green bell pepper, cored, seeded, and thinly sliced

   1 small yam, peeled and shredded, about 1 cup

   1 carrot, peeled and shredded, about ½ cup

Fresh chives for garnish

....

Dressing

4 Tbsp cider vinegar or apple cider

3 Tbsp fresh lime juice or more to taste

1 tsp honey

2/3 cups extra-virgin olive oil

Kosher salt and freshly ground pepper to taste

1. Cut cabbages in half, quarter, remove core. Thinly slice with sharp knife on diagonal. Mix together the cabbage, peppers, yams, and carrots in large bowl.

2. In small bowl combine dressing ingredients and whisk until well combined. Adjust seasoning to taste.

3. Toss with cabbage mixture and chill for several hours to meld flavors. When ready to serve, garnish with fresh chives.

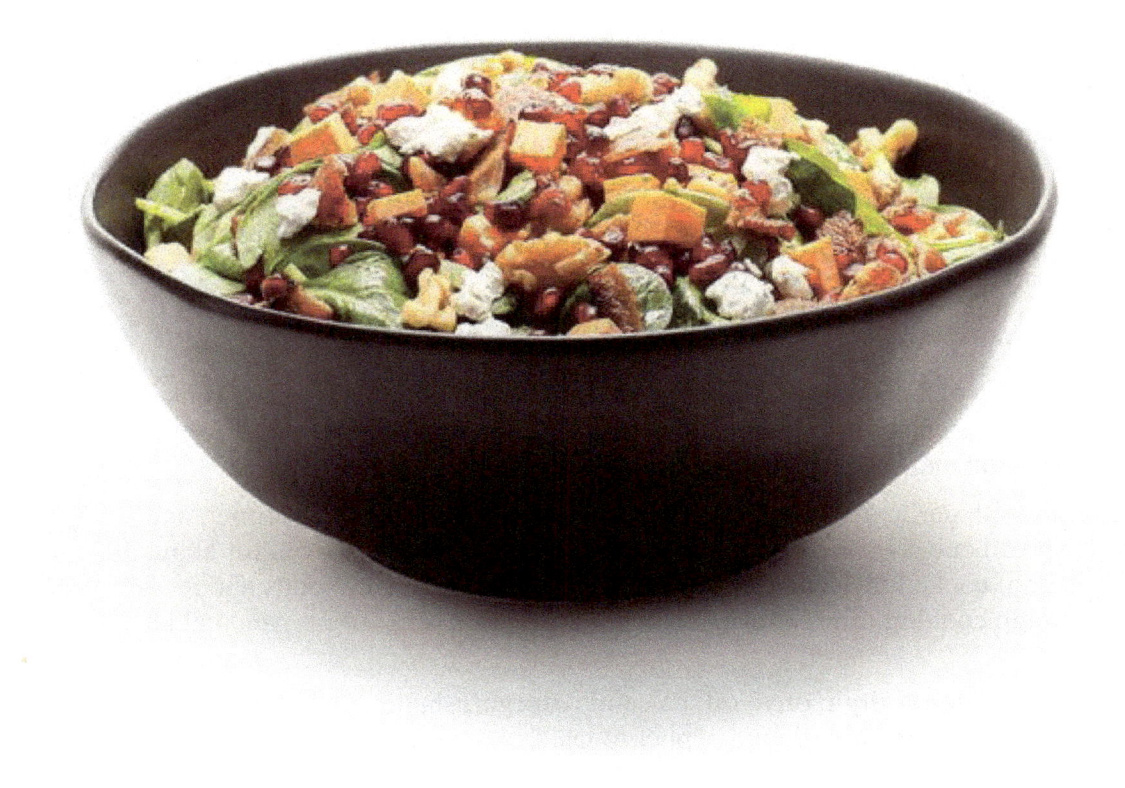

Spinach Salad with Sweet Potato, Bacon, Walnuts, and Pomegranates

This bountiful salad fills every bite with new tastes. Pomegranates provide little explosions of flavor that give this salad a respite from the ordinary.

Serves 8

    16 oz nitrate-free bacon

    1 medium yam, washed, peeled, cut into ½-inch cubes, about 2 cups

    Pinch of garlic salt

    Pinch of ground cinnamon

    Pinch of ground ginger

    Pinch of Kosher salt and freshly ground pepper

18–24 ounces baby spinach, washed and dried

¼ cup Gruyere, grated or your favorite cheese

A few handfuls of pomegranate seeds

A handful of whole walnuts

5 Tbsp extra-virgin olive oil

3 Tbsp balsamic vinegar

1 shallot, diced

½ tsp Grey Poupon

Ground sea salt and freshly ground pepper to taste

....

1. Preheat oven to 425 degrees with rack in the center. In a large frying pan, cook bacon until brown and crispy. Remove from pan and drain on paper towel. Reserve 1 teaspoon bacon fat and set aside to cool. Crumble bacon.

2. Toss cubes with garlic salt, cinnamon, ginger, ground sea salt, black pepper, and bacon fat. Spread cubes on a cookie sheet in a single layer. Roast in oven for about 30-35 minutes until cooked through and golden brown. Turn once with tongs about halfway through cooking time for even browning. Remove yams from oven and let cool.

3. Whisk together extra-virgin olive oil, balsamic vinegar, shallot, and Grey Poupon mustard. Add salt and freshly ground pepper to taste.

4. Place baby spinach in a large bowl. Top with bacon crumbles, roasted yams, Gruyere, pomegranate seeds, and walnuts. Toss with vinaigrette.

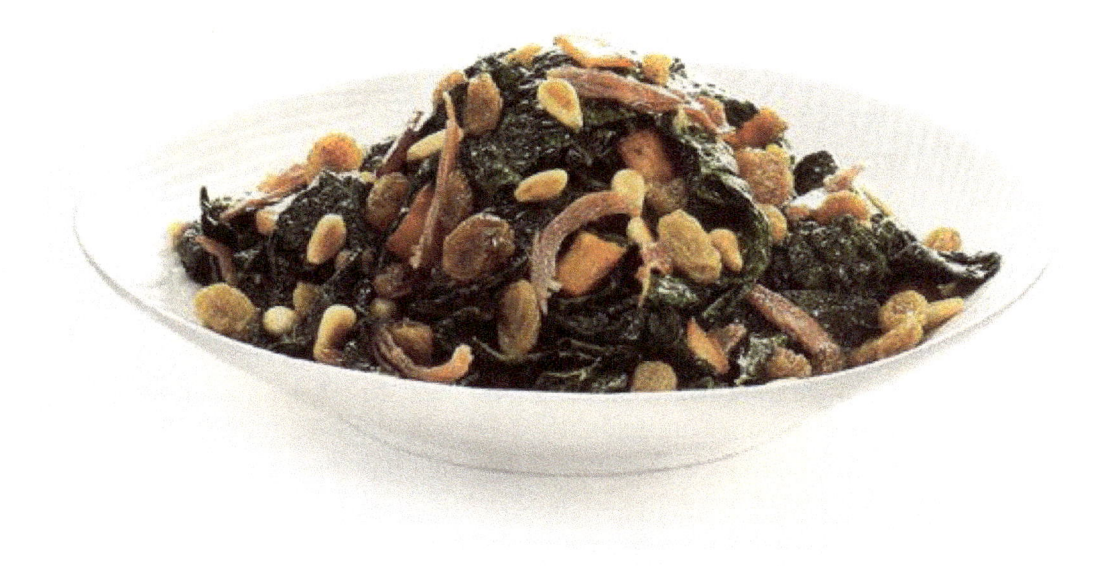

Chard with Sweet Potato, Pine Nuts, Golden Raisins, and Prosciutto

All green, leafy goodness should taste as good as this. The mingling of flavors and textures make every bite a tasting adventure of what pops out next.

Serves 6

¾ cup golden raisins

¼ star anise

1 whole clove

½ cup dry white wine

2 Tbsp pine nuts

3 oz thinly sliced prosciutto, cut crosswise into ¼-inch strips

4 Tbsp extra-virgin olive oil

1 small yam, peeled, cut into ½-inch cubes, about 1 cup

Kosher salt and freshly ground black pepper

1 bunch chard or kale

1 Tbsp garlic, finely chopped

....

1. Combine the golden raisins, star anise, and clove in a small jar. In a small saucepan, bring the wine to a boil. Pour over the raisins and cool. Let stand for 30 minutes. (Covered, raisin mixture can be refrigerated for up to one month.) Remove the star anise and clove before using.

2. In a large sauté pan on medium-high heat, brown pine nuts (2–3 minutes), shaking to brown evenly. Remove to plate and cool. In same pan add the prosciutto and sauté for about a minute to crisp. Remove to bowl. In the same pan, heat 2 tablespoons of oil over medium heat and sauté yam cubes until slightly browned, about 5 minutes (but hold their shape). Salt and pepper to taste. Remove to bowl with prosciutto.

3. Cut the thick stems from the kale or chard and discard. Stack the greens in batches and cut crosswise into 1-inch strips. Set aside. Add 1½ tablespoons oil into the pan and heat over medium-low heat. Add the garlic and cook until softened but not brown, about 1 minute. Add one half the chard greens, season with salt and pepper, cook 3–5 minutes over medium-low to medium heat, until the chard wilts to about half its original volume. Add remaining chard and cook until wilted and tender, 5–10 minutes.

4. Add pine nuts to bowl with yams and prosciutto. Add 2-3 tablespoons of raisins with their liquid and toss. Season to taste with salt and pepper. Add to pan with the greens, toss and serve.

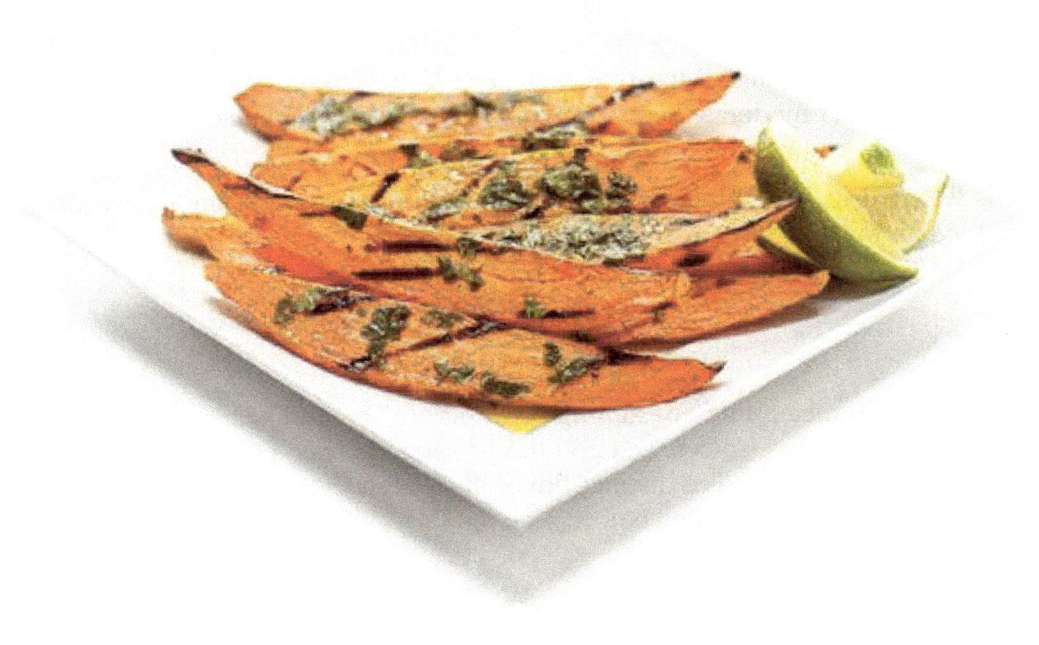

Grilled Sweet Potato with Lime and Cilantro Dressing

Crispy on the outside and chewy on the inside, these sweet potato wedges are a tasty treat. Lime cilantro dressing gives them a kick. The tartness is a surprisingly good combination to accompany the sweetness.

Serves 8

- 4 medium yams, about the same size
- 1/3 cup lime juice, 3-4 limes
- 1½ tsp Kosher salt
- ¼ tsp freshly ground black pepper
- ½ cup extra-virgin olive oil
- ¼ cup chopped cilantro, reserve 1 tsp for garnish
- 1 lime, quartered

1. In a large pot, cover yams with cold salted water. Bring to a boil. Simmer until slightly resistant when pierced (about 20–25 minutes). Place in large bowl of ice water to stop cooking. When cool, drain. Peel yams and quarter lengthwise.

2. Whisk together lime juice, salt, and pepper, and add oil in slow stream, whisking. Whisk in cilantro. Taste to adjust seasoning.

3. Heat and lightly oil grill. When hot, place yams on grill, uncovered. Turn when grill marks appear, about 2–3 minutes. Repeat on each side. Yams can also be cooked on an oiled-ridged grill pan over moderate heat, turning when grill marks appear and just tender.

4. Serve yams warm, drizzled with dressing. Garnish with lime quarters and reserved cilantro sprinkled on top.

Sweet Potato Mash Three Ways

Great flavor does not have to mean time-consuming preparation. Oven-baked sweet potatoes can be jazzed up with different proteins, spices, and goodies to keep interest. Try experimenting with the varieties of sweet potatoes. Each has a distinct flavor that is fun to explore. Sweet potato mash can be made the day ahead and heated before serving.

Sweet Potato Prep

Serves 8

Preheat oven to 400 degrees. Arrange yams on a baking sheet lined with aluminum foil. Bake 1 hour or until easily pierced with a fork. Remove from oven and let stand until cool enough to handle.

....

Mashed Sweet Potato with Orange and Ginger

4 medium sweet potatoes, baked

Juice of one orange or to taste

1 tsp orange rind, grated

1 tsp lemon rind, grated

1 tsp fresh ginger root, grated

Pinch of ground nutmeg

2–3 Tbsp organic maple syrup or to taste

1. Scoop out flesh. Purée flesh in food processor with remaining ingredients. Adjust seasoning. Place mixture in ovenproof bowl, cover, and heat in a 350-degree oven for 15 minutes or until heated through.

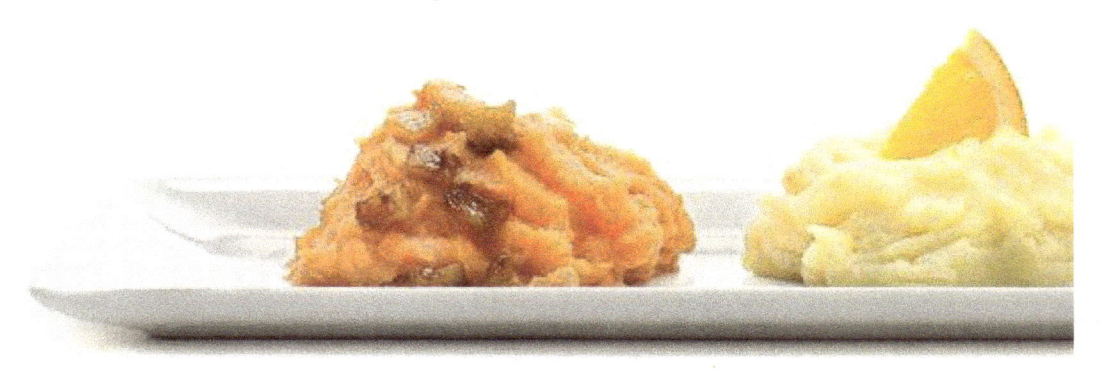

Okinawa Mash

4 Okinawa sweet potatoes, baked

4 Tbsp butter, melted

Kosher salt and pepper

1. Scoop out flesh. Purée flesh in food processor with butter. Salt and pepper to taste. Put mixture in ovenproof bowl, cover, and heat in a 350-degree oven for 15 minutes or until heated through.

....

Whipped Yams with Caramelized Apples

4 medium yams, baked

¼ cup unsalted butter, melted

2 Tbsp heavy cream

½ cup applesauce

2 tsp fresh peeled ginger, grated

1 tsp Kosher salt

Freshly ground pepper

2 apples, peeled, cored, and cut into ½-inch chunks

1 Tbsp honey

1. Scoop out flesh. Purée flesh in food processor with butter, cream, applesauce, and ginger. Salt and pepper to taste. Put mixture in ovenproof bowl, cover, and heat in a 350-degree oven for 15 minutes or until heated through.

2. Meanwhile, toss apples with honey in a bowl. In a small sauté pan, heat mixture on medium. Sauté until apples are slightly brown and honey has evaporated, about 3-5 minutes. Remove yams from oven; top with caramelized apples and serve.

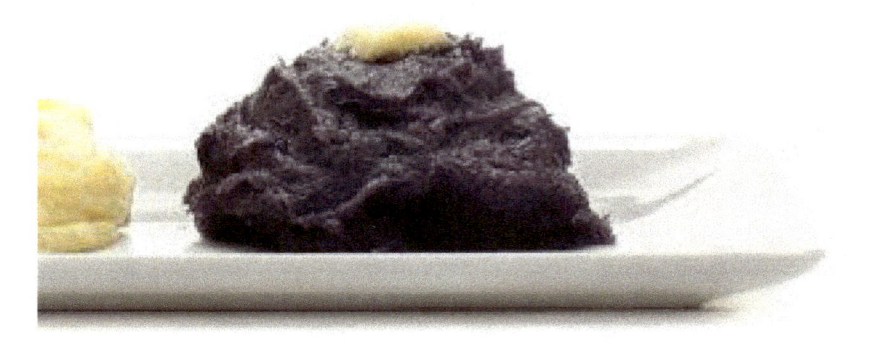

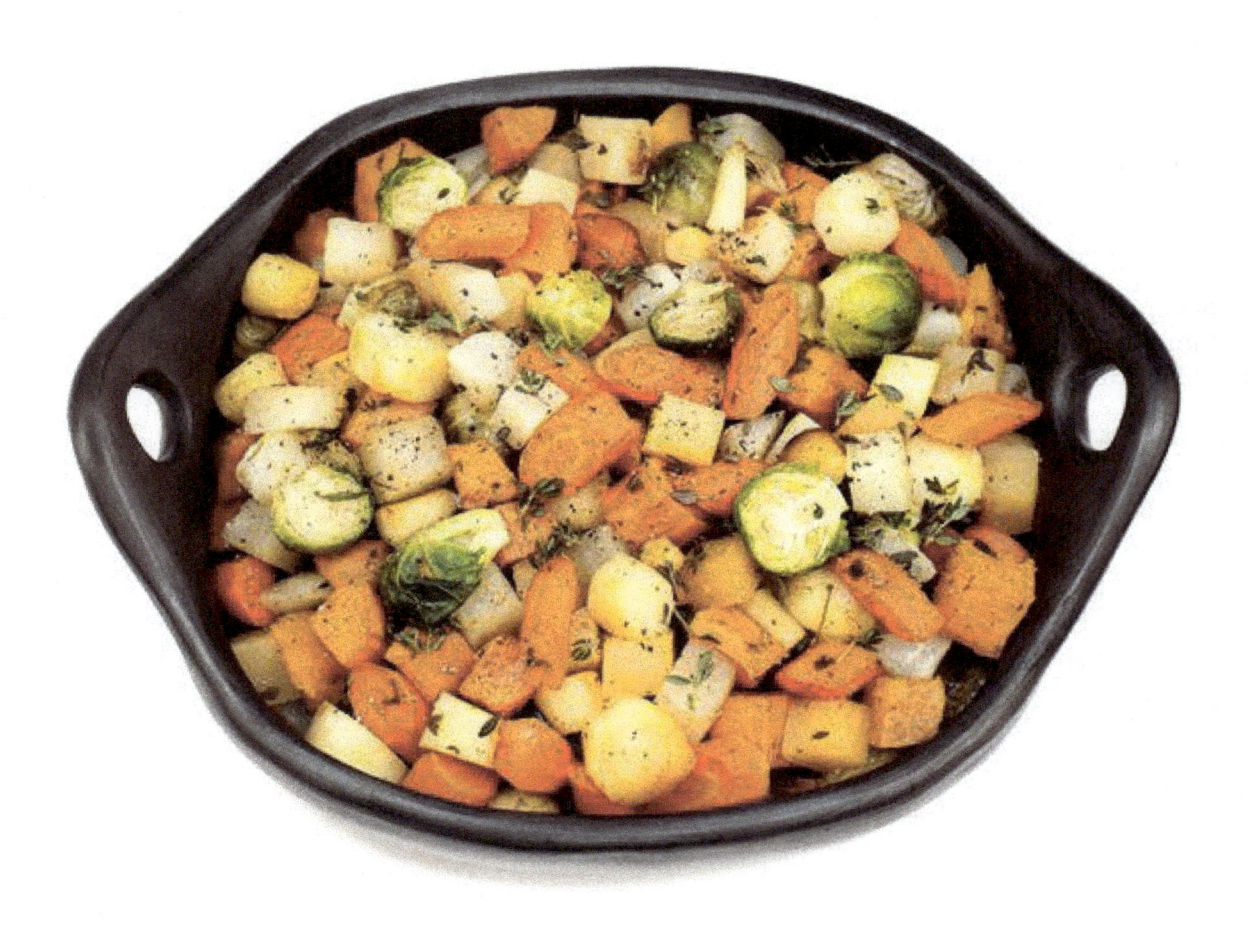

Oven-Roasted Winter Vegetables

Great dishes do not have to be complicated, and this medley is as simple as it gets. Although humble in origin, the merits of these roasted roots speak for themselves with earthy goodness.

Serves 8

- ¾ lb small-in-diameter organic yams, washed and cut into 1-inch pieces (leave peel on)
- ¾ lb carrots, peeled and cut into 1-inch pieces
- ¾ lbs Brussels sprouts, trimmed and cut in half
- ¾ lb rutabagas, peeled and cut into 1-inch pieces
- ¾ lb parsnips, peeled and cut into 1-inch pieces
- 1½ Tbsp unsalted butter
- 1½ Tbsp extra-virgin olive oil
- 1 Tbsp fresh thyme, finely chopped
- 1 Tbsp ground sage, finely chopped
- 1 tsp ground nutmeg
- Kosher salt and freshly ground black pepper

....

1. Preheat oven to 450 degrees. Place the vegetables in a large roasting pan.

2. In a small saucepan, melt butter and stir in the olive oil, thyme, sage, and nutmeg. Drizzle the butter mixture over the vegetables and toss to coat. Season to taste with salt and pepper.

3. Cover vegetables with foil and roast for 30 minutes. Remove the foil, toss the vegetables and continue to cook until the vegetables can be easily pierced with a knife, about 15–20 minutes. Place the roasted vegetables on a platter and serve.

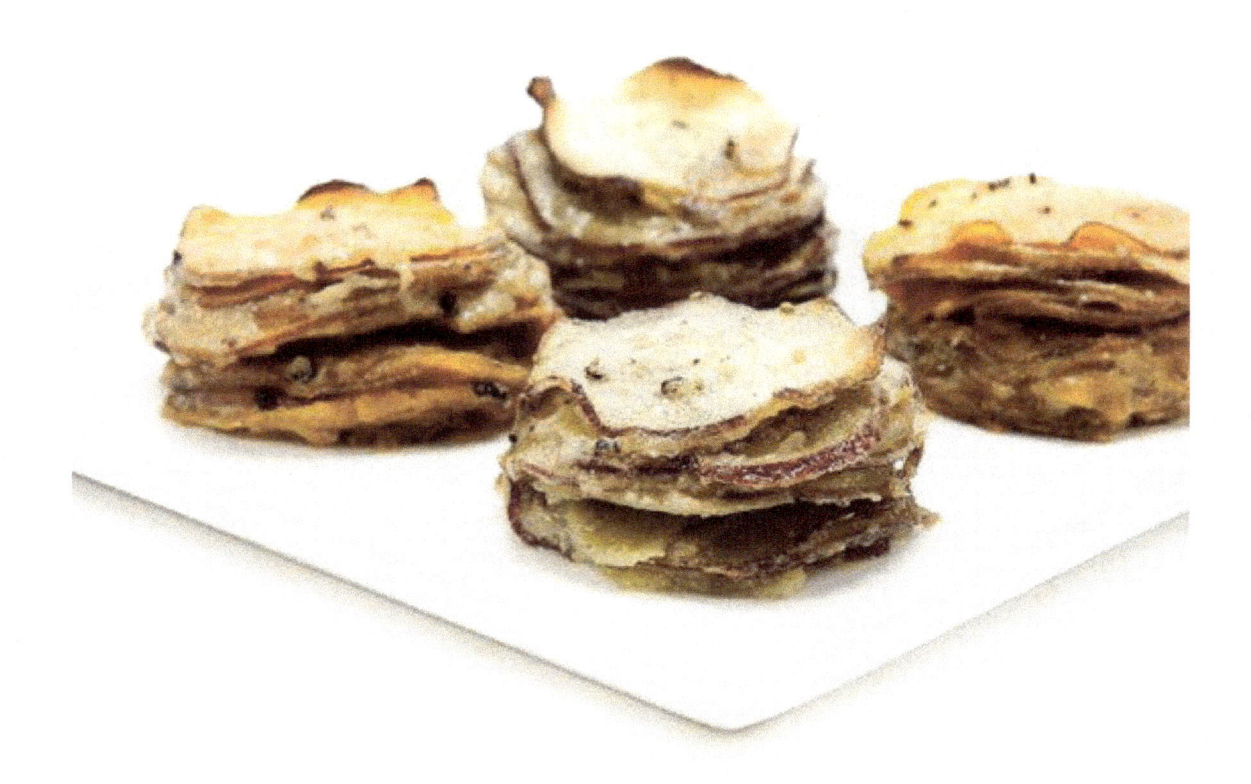

Sweet Potato Gratin Stackers

Gratins speak to the food soul. The hot, gooey, rich, stacked, sweet potato baked in a muffin tin is a more indulgent treat than usual vegetable sides. Their flavors mingle and meld in a dish that is effortless to make.

Serves 6

> 2 medium sweet potatoes (one white sweet potato and one yam), no fatter than muffin tin, peeled and sliced crosswise on the mandoline, keep the white and yams separate
>
> Kosher salt and freshly ground pepper to taste
>
> 1 cup of heavy cream
>
> Unsalted butter for brushing muffin cups

....

> 1. Preheat oven to 400 degrees. Lightly brush a 6-cup muffin pan with butter.
>
> 2. Beginning with the yams, place two slices in each cup and season with salt and pepper. Continue adding slices, seasoning every few slices, until the cups are filled. Continue filling muffin cups with the white sweet potatoes slices.

3. Pour 1–2 tablespoons of heavy cream over each, allowing cream to drip down the sides. Bake until the sweet potatoes are golden brown and tender when pierced with a knife, about 30–35 minutes.

4. Run a knife around each gratin. Place a large plate over pan and invert to release gratins. Flip right side up and serve hot.

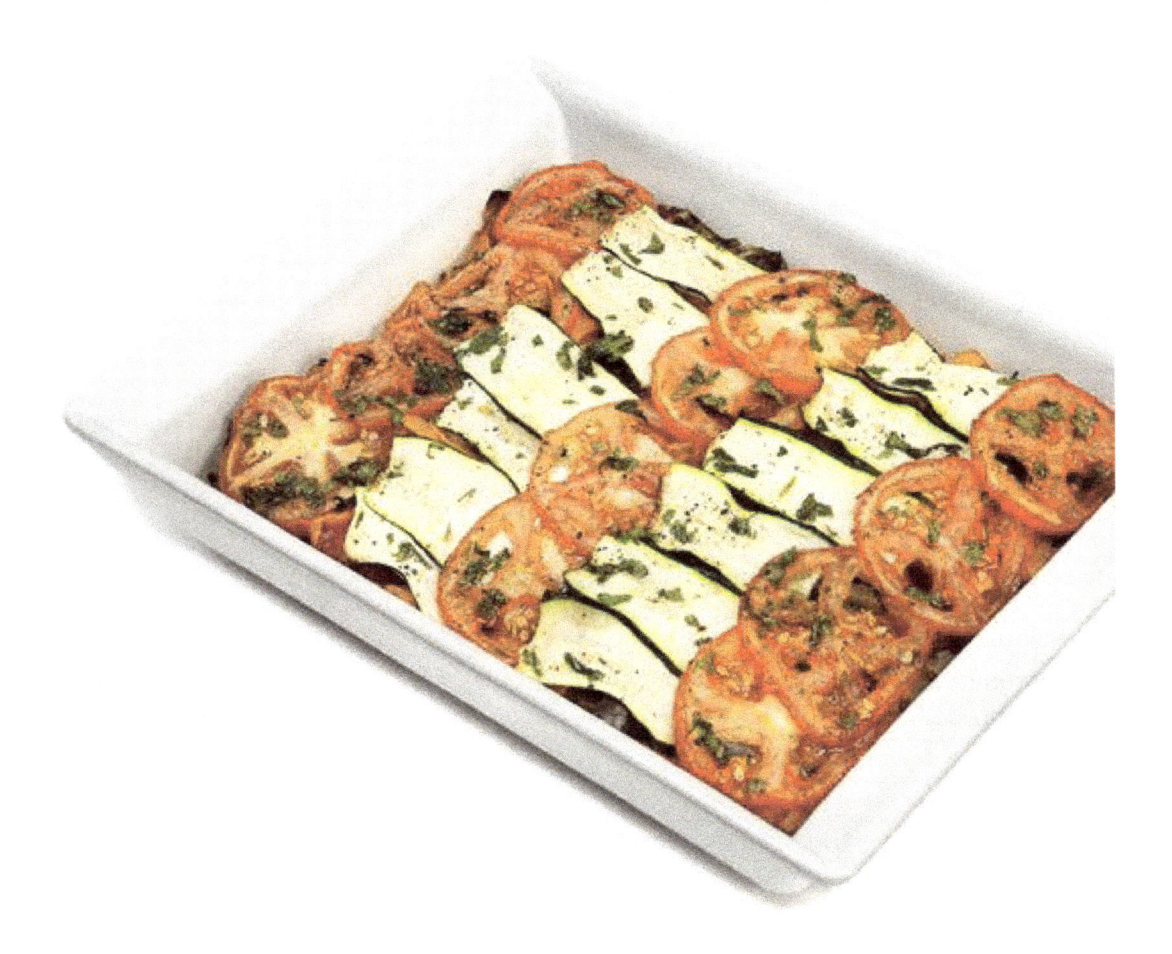

Vegetable Tian

This casserole is full of flavorful veggies. Tians are a homey specialty of Provence made from seasonal vegetables. Variations abound. Don't be afraid to add whatever veggies you might have. Use the recipe as a base and experiment by adding your favorite goodies.

Serves 6

- 4 Tbsp extra-virgin olive oil
- 2 onions, peeled and thinly sliced

1 red bell pepper, rib removed, seeded, and thinly sliced

1 green bell pepper, rib removed, seeded, and thinly sliced

1 small yam, peeled and thinly sliced lengthwise on mandoline and cut into ¼-inch strips

1 small eggplant, thinly sliced, cut into ¼-inch strips

4–6 garlic cloves, chopped

2 tsp or more chopped fresh herbs: marjoram, thyme, rosemary, Italian parsley, mixed together

Kosher salt and freshly ground pepper

2 lbs young, tender zucchini, cut into thin slices

2 lbs medium ripe tomatoes, cut into thin slices

4 Tbsp flat-leaf parsley, finely cut

....

1. Preheat oven to 375 degrees. In large sauté pan, heat 2 tablespoons of oil to medium. Lightly sauté the onions, peppers, yam, and eggplant. When softened, add half of the garlic and cook a few minutes longer. Season to taste with half of the herbs, salt, and pepper.

2. Place sautéed vegetables in baking dish. On top arrange the sliced zucchini and tomatoes in overlapping rows so that you see stripes of white-green, red, white-green, red, etc. Sprinkle the top with salt, pepper, the remaining herbs, garlic, parsley, and drizzle with remaining olive oil. Bake for 30–40 minutes, until top is slightly browned. Garnish with parsley. Serve.

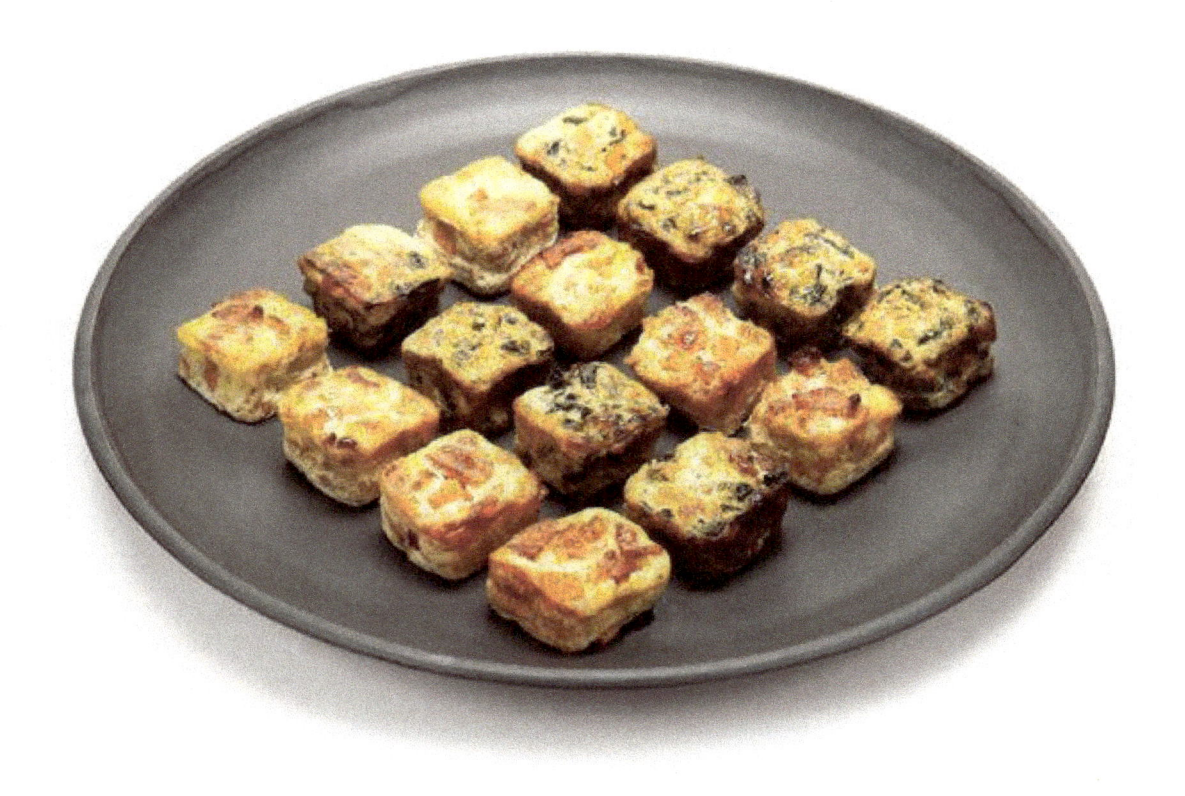

On-the-Go Sweet Potato Quiche

Good clean, on-the-go protein is hard to come by. These little gems are great for lunch and snacks because they don't make a mess if they get smushed in a bag. They're also easy to make and hold up without refrigeration for a short period of time.

Makes 24 mini-bites

    1 leek, white and light green, quartered and sliced, about 1 cup

    ½ cup water

    1 tsp Kosher salt

    1 tsp unsalted butter

    6 slices bacon, nitrate-free, cut into ½-inch pieces

    3 eggs

    1½ cups half-and-half

    Couple pinches of nutmeg

    Kosher salt and freshly ground pepper to taste

    1 medium yam, baked until done but still slightly firm, peeled and cut into ½-inch pieces

¼ cup Gruyere cheese, grated

1 cup spinach, steamed (optional)

Coconut oil spray for coating

1 Tbsp unsalted butter, cut in pea-size dots

....

1. Heat oven to 375 degrees. In a small saucepan, boil water and add the leeks, salt, and butter. Cook over medium heat, covered, until water has almost evaporated. Lower heat and stew gently for 10-15 minutes or until tender.

2. In small frying pan, on medium heat add bacon pieces and cook until crisp. In mixing bowl beat together the eggs, cream, and seasonings. Check the seasoning. Gently add the diced yam, bacon pieces, and cheese.

3. Spray mini-muffin pan with coconut oil spray. Place about a tablespoon of the quiche mixture in each cup. Top with pea-size piece of butter. Bake for 20 minutes or until golden on top. Remove from oven, cool for 10 minutes, and remove from pan to cooling rack.

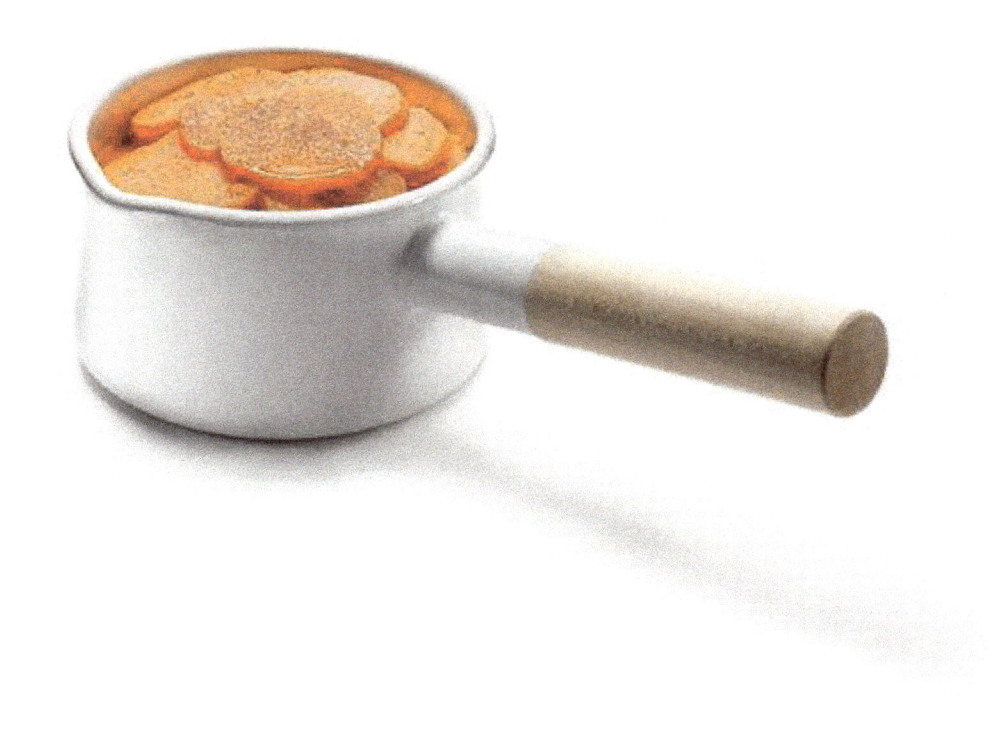

Spicy Sliced Sweet Potato

No need for sides to be boring. Spicy Sliced Sweet Potato will make your taste buds dance. Full of Eastern flavors, this side can be ready in minutes.

Serves 4

- 1 medium yam, narrow not fat, peeled and thinly sliced, about 2 cups
- 1 cup fresh orange juice (fresh makes a difference)
- ¼ cup water
- ½ tsp ground coriander
- ½ tsp ground cumin
- ¼ tsp ground cinnamon
- 1 Tbsp unsalted butter
- Kosher salt

....

1. In a medium saucepan of boiling salted water, blanch the yam slices for 1 minute. Drain and set aside.

2. In the same pan, combine the orange juice, water, coriander, cumin, and cinnamon. Add the yams and simmer over moderate heat, stirring occasionally, until just tender, about 3-5 minutes.

3. Remove from saucepan and stir in butter. Season with salt to taste. Serve.

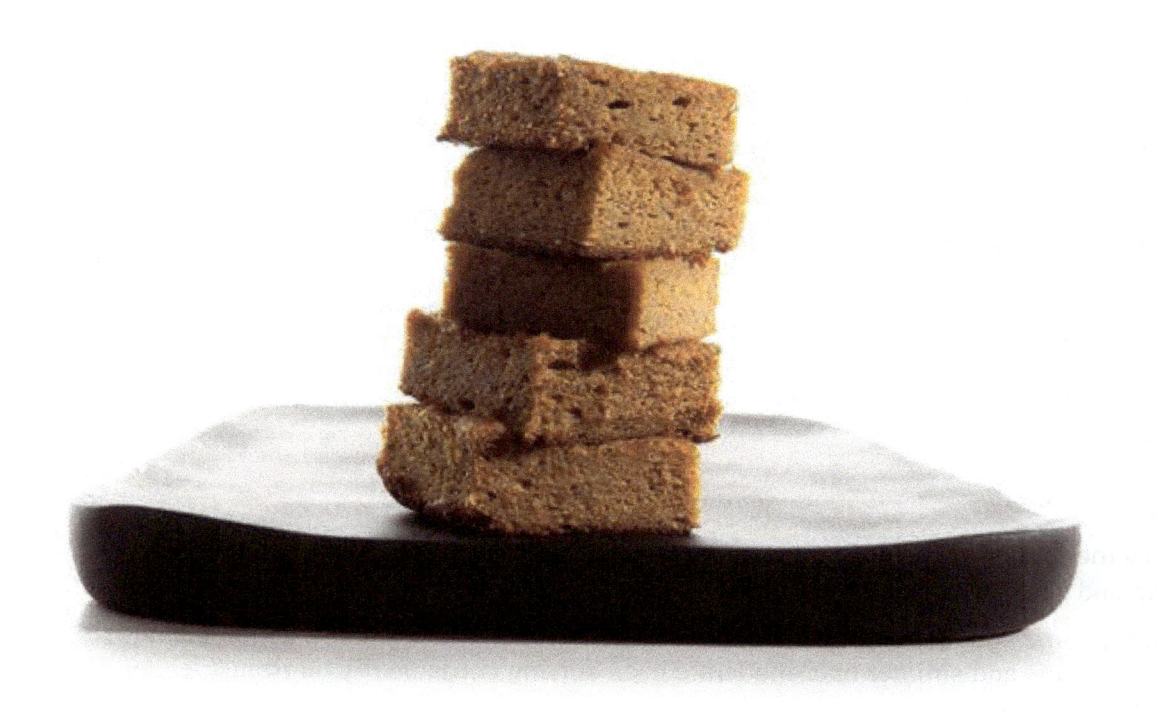

Sweet Potato Bars

Flourless cake recipes should be as good or better than wheat flour counterparts. Sweet Potato Bars rise above their inspiration. Moist, filling, finger-licking good, they taste like pumpkin pie and have none of the guilt. Make them year-rouncd for a new comfort-food staple.

Serves 9

½ cup yam purée

1/3 cup honey

2 eggs

1 cup blanched almond flour

¼ tsp ground sea salt

½ tsp baking soda

¼ tsp cinnamon

¼ tsp nutmeg

¼ tsp cloves

....

1. To make purée: Heat oven to 400 degrees. Place medium yam on baking sheet and bake for 1 hour or until easily pierced with a fork. Cool, scoop out flesh from skin. Discard skin. Purée flesh in food processor. (Mash can be made days ahead and frozen or refrigerated until ready to use.)

2. For bars: Heat oven to 350 degrees. In a food processor, combine purée, honey, and eggs. Pulse for 2 minutes. Add dry flour and seasonings. Pulse for a full minute.

3. Pour batter into a greased, 8-inch square baking dish. Bake for 30–35 minutes. Serve.

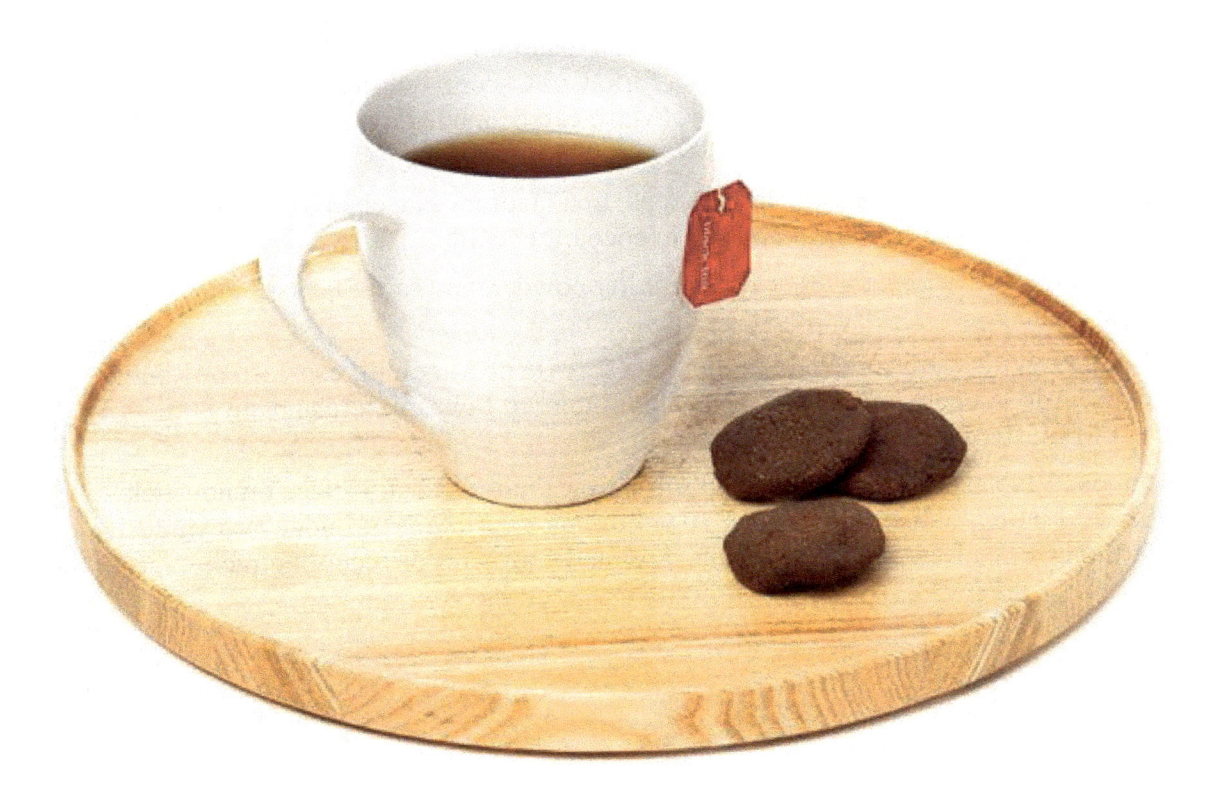

Fudge Brownie Bites

Pure, fudgy, chocolaty goodness, these brownie bites are rich and decedent. It's a dessert that is sure to satisfy and make you wonder why anyone bothers with wheat.

Serves 24

    2/3 cup yam purée

4 Tbsp (½ stick) unsalted butter

2/3 cup natural unsweetened cocoa powder

½ cup coconut flour

¼ tsp baking powder

¼ tsp sea salt

2/3 cup honey

1 large egg, beaten

1½ tsp vanilla extract

½ tsp instant espresso powder

....

1. To make purée: Heat oven to 400 degrees. Place medium yam on baking sheet and bake for 1 hour or until easily pierced with a fork. Cool, scoop out flesh from skin. Discard skin. Purée flesh in food processor. (Mash can be made days ahead and frozen or refrigerated until ready to use.)

2. For Brownie Bites: Heat oven to 350 degrees. In a medium saucepan over low heat, melt butter. Remove pan from heat and stir in cocoa. Let cool.

3. In a medium bowl, whisk together flour, baking powder, and salt. Stir in honey, sweet potato, and egg.

4. In a small prep dish, stir together vanilla and espresso powder until espresso powder is dissolved. Add to cocoa mixture. Add cocoa mixture to flour mixture and stir until no traces of flour remain.

5. Take about 1 tablespoon of mixture and roll into walnut-size balls. Place on nonstick cookie sheet. Flatten to disk shape. Bake 10–15 minutes until tops of Fudge Brownie Bites start to crackle. Remove from baking sheet and cool bites on a cooling rack.

Chocolate Sweet Potato Truffles

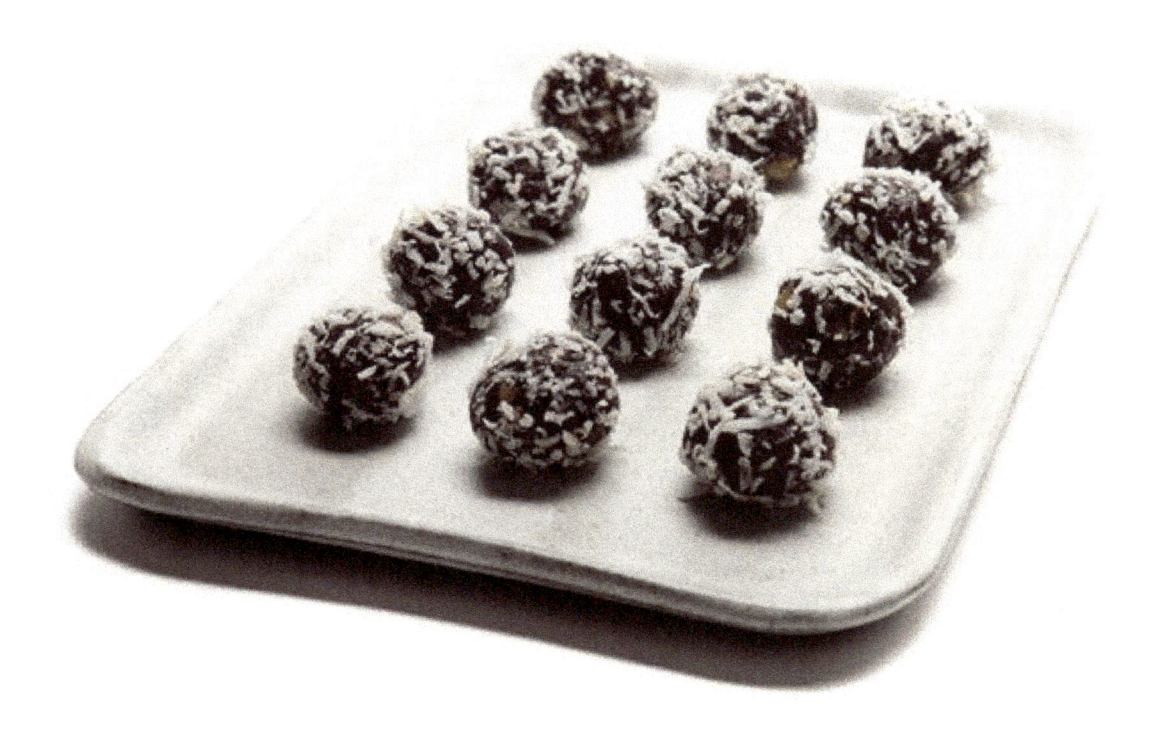

Life at times calls for a little bite of something special. Chocolate Sweet Potato Truffles are made with nature's goodness. Rich and decadent, they hit the spot when the sweet tooth calls. Freeze to enjoy one at a time or share with friends.

Makes 24 small truffles

- 1/3 cup of Okinawa sweet potato (purple) purée
- 15 pitted Medjool dates
- 1½ cups raw walnuts
- ½ cup of raw cacao
- ½ cup of raw, unsweetened, shredded coconut (optional)

....

1. To make purée: Heat oven to 400 degrees. Place Okinawa sweet potato on baking sheet and bake for 1 hour or until easily pierced with a fork. Cool, scoop out flesh from skin. Discard skin. Purée flesh in food processor. (Mash can be made days ahead, refrigerated until ready to use.)

2. Remove pits from dates, set aside. Chop ¼ cup walnuts, set aside.

3. In a food processor, place remaining 1¼ cup of walnuts. Grind until fine. Add medjool dates and mashed sweet potato. Blend until walnuts and dates stick together. Add raw cacao. Blend until incorporated.

4. Remove mixture from food processor. Fold in chopped walnuts until incorporated evenly. Take a teaspoon-size amount and roll gently between palms into a ball. Roll balls in coconut shavings.

5. Place on a tray. Refrigerate until set, at least an hour. Enjoy immediately or freeze.

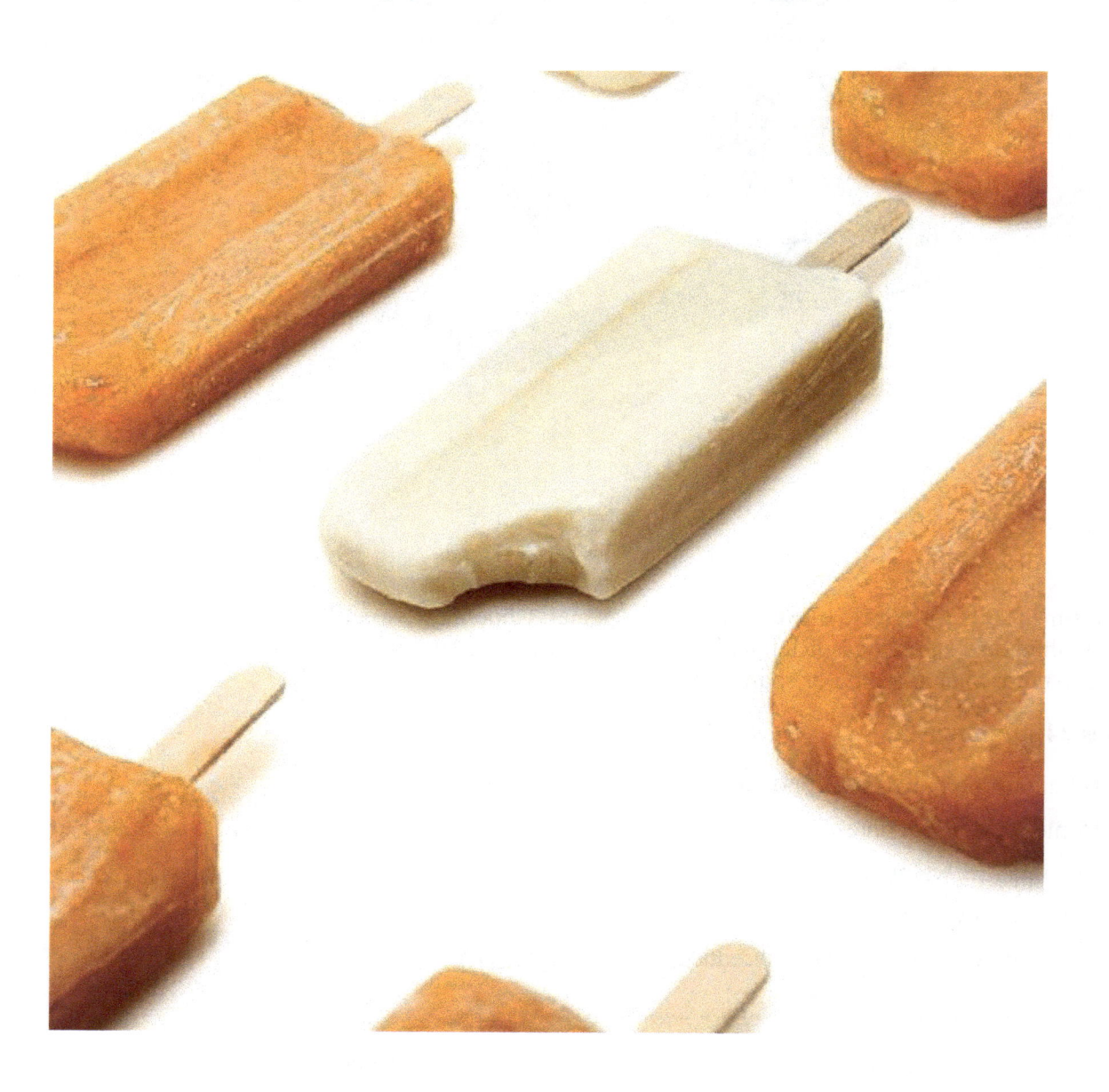

Sweet Potato Ice Pops

Pops are fun but often loaded with sugar. Sweet-potato pops are a nutritious and less sweet alternative. Flavor and color make these treats perfect for summer days or to ward off the ice cream boogie monster. Kids and adults alike will not know this pop is so good for them.

Serves 6

    1 cup mashed Satsumaimo sweet potato or yam

    1 can coconut milk

    ½ can (6 oz) of pineapple concentrate

    ½ tsp salt

    1 tsp orange zest

....

1. To make purée: Heat oven to 400 degrees. Place medium Satsumaimo sweet potato or yam on baking sheet and bake for 1 hour or until easily pierced with a fork. Cool, scoop out flesh from skin. Discard skin. Purée flesh in food processor. (Mash can be made days ahead and refrigerated until ready to use.)

2. Place 1 cup mash and remaining ingredients in blender. Cover and blend 10–15 seconds or until smooth. Pour into pop molds and freeze until solid, about 4 hours.

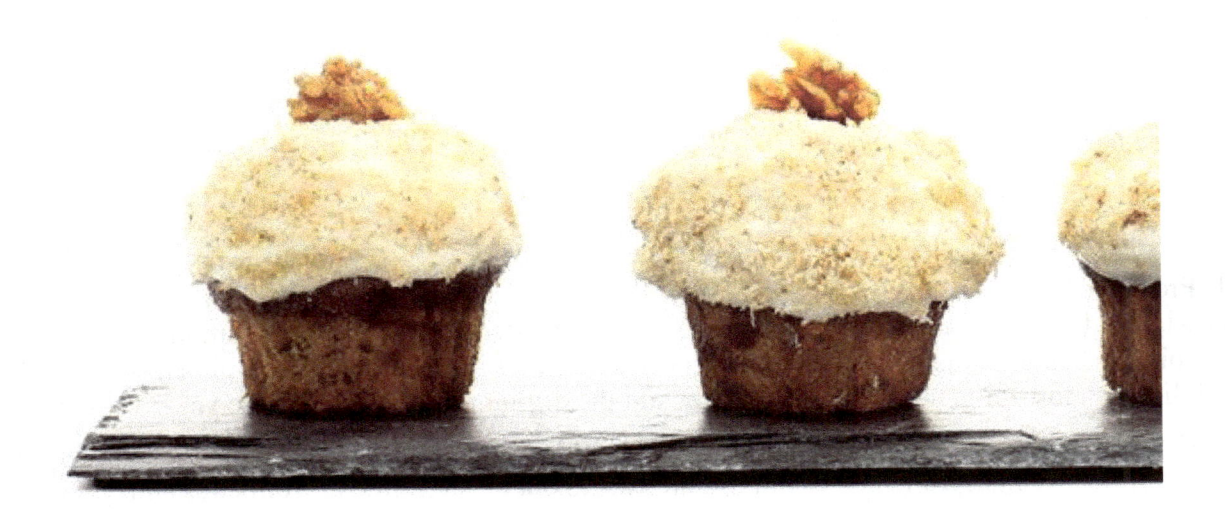

Sweet Potato Cupcakes

Special treats have a place in life. Not every day, not even every week, but on special occasions, they can be just what the doctor ordered. Some foods are worth the splurge. These cupcakes are one of them, while also being a "better cheat."

Servings 12 cupcakes

- 1 cup gluten-free flour, like C4C
- ¼ cup almond meal
- ½ tsp baking powder
- ½ tsp baking soda
- 1 tsp ground cinnamon
- ¼ tsp allspice
- ¼ tsp salt
- ¼ whole milk
- 2 eggs
- 1/3 cup coconut oil, melted
- 2/3 cup honey
- 1 tsp pure vanilla extract
- 1 small yam, peeled and shredded (about 1 cup)
- 6-oz of cream cheese, room temp
- ¼ cup unsalted butter, melted
- ½ cup powdered sugar, sifted
- ½ tsp vanilla extract

1. Preheat oven to 350 degrees. Line 12 cupcake cups with paper liners. In a large bowl, mix together the flour, almond meal, baking powder, baking soda, cinnamon, allspice and salt. Set aside. In the bowl of a mixer fitted with a paddle, beat milk, eggs, oil, honey and vanilla until smooth. Slowly add the dry ingredients. Mix in the yam.

2. Divide the batter among the lined cupcake cups. Bake for 20 minutes or until wooden skewer inserted in center of cupcake comes out clean. Remove from cups and cool to room temperature on a cooling rack.

3. Meanwhile, in small saucepan, melt butter and slightly cool. In a clean bowl of a stand mixer fitted with the paddle, beat the cream cheese at medium speed until smooth. Add the butter to cream cheese and mix until smooth. Beat in powdered sugar, add vanilla. Scrape down sides and beat for 30 seconds on high speed until smooth.

4. Spread tops of the cupcakes with the cream cheese frosting and sprinkle with chopped walnuts. Although best eaten the day they are baked, they can be frozen.

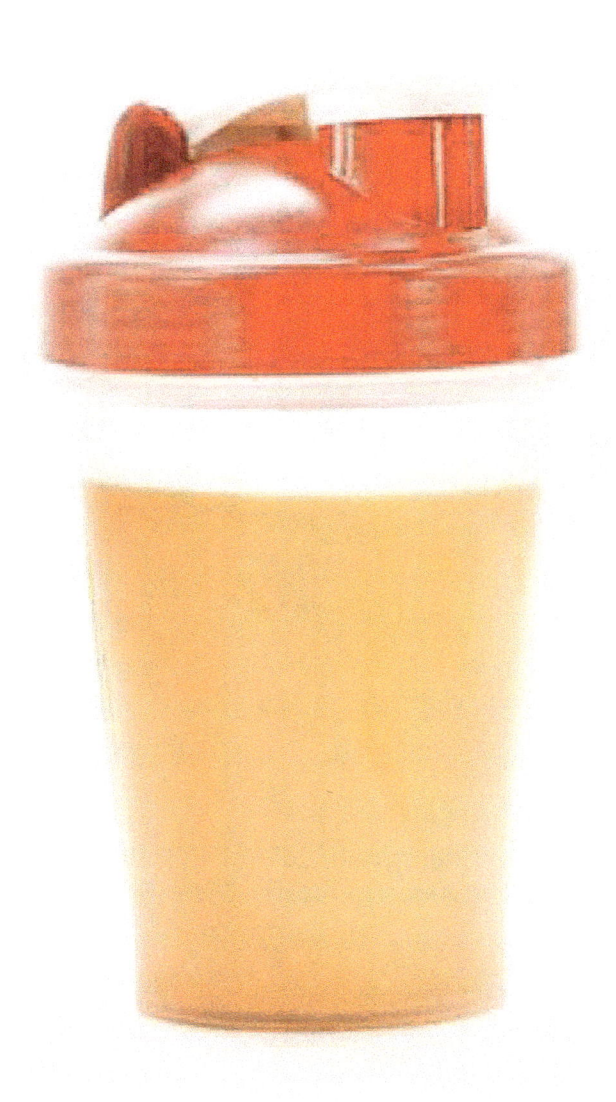

Recovery Drink

Note: If you are trying to lean out, this shake is not for you. Stick to protein until you have reached your desired weight, then smartly add carbs back into your diet.

This post-workout shake is full of good carbs and protein to aid recovery. Timing is everything. Prep ahead and freeze in batches. The recovery drink should be consumed in the prime window, 15–30 minutes after a hard workout. Use the recipe as a guide and don't be afraid to add favorite supplements.

Serves 1

- ½ cup sweet potato mash
- 1 cup whole milk
- 2 egg whites
- 1/8 tsp ground cinnamon
- 1 pinch ground nutmeg
- 1 pinch ginger
- 1 pinch allspice
- Optional supplements:
- Branch chain amino acids (BCAA)
- L-glutamine
- R-lipoic acid (R-ALA)

1. To make mash: Heat oven to 400 degrees. Place medium yam on baking sheet and bake for 1 hour or until easily pierced with a fork. Cool, scoop out flesh from skin. Discard skin. Purée flesh in food processor.

2. Put all ingredients in a blender and blend till smooth. If you are uncomfortable with consuming raw eggs, consider experimenting with Eggology. Place shake in a recovery container and shake before drinking. Do your own research before starting a new supplement program.

....

About the Supplements

Branch chain amino acids (BCAA): Hard and long training causes the breakdown of muscles. BCAA helps blunt the effects of a hard workout, protecting the muscles from breakdown.

L-glutamine has been found to help with muscle recovery when training hard and to have immune-stimulating properties. Supplement with 10 grams post-workout.

R-lipoic acid (R-ALA) helps improve insulin sensitivity and has antioxidant effects. It also plays an important role in recharging vitamin C and E stores. Take 200–500 mg daily

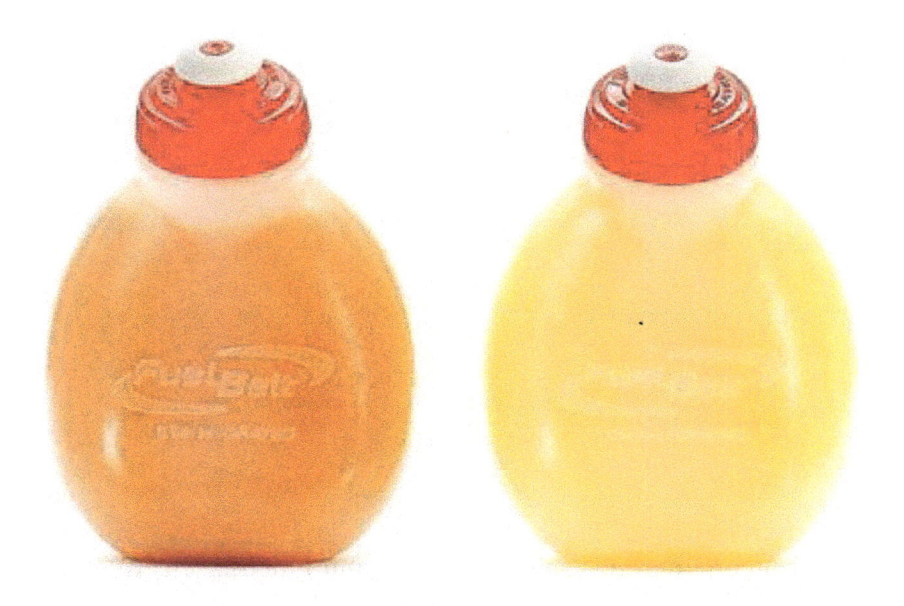

Sport Gels Three Ways

Forgo the fructose and make your own octane. Sport gels are an excellent way to keep real food the foundation of your diet while at the same time avoiding crashes and sugar spikes mid-race. They are easy to make, freeze like a dream, and will become a staple for your big days out. Add protein powder or egg whites for extended activity over an hour.

Serves 2

....

Tropical

- 1 cup yam mash
- ½ cup coconut milk
- 1 cup orange juice
- Juice of one lime
- Juice of one lemon
- Pinch of salt

Apple Cinnamon

- 1 cup yam mash
- 1 cup apple cider
- 1 cup hazelnut milk
- 1 pinch cinnamon
- 1 pinch cloves
- 1 pinch salt

Lime Aid

- 1 cup Satsumaimo sweet potato mash
- ¼ coconut milk
- 2 cups orange juice
- Zest of one orange
- 1 pinch of salt

Note: If you are trying to lean out, use gels sparingly until your glucose sensitivity returns, and you reach your desired weight. Then add them in smartly to fuel extended intense physical activity or races.

1. To make mash: Heat oven to 400 degrees. Place medium yam or Satsumaimo sweet potato on baking sheet and bake for 1 hour or until easily pierced with a fork. Cool, scoop out flesh from skin. Discard skin. Purée flesh in food processor. (Mash can be made days ahead and refrigerated until ready to use.)

2. Place ingredients in blender and blend until smooth. If batter is too thick, add extra liquid.

3. Pour into sports gel containers found at sports stores. Use immediately or freeze.